Gender
Transition

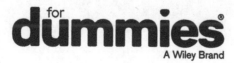

Gender Transition

by Adrien Lawyer, T. Michael Trimm, Erik Wolf, and Molly McClain, MD MPH MS

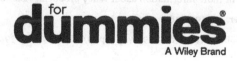

Gender Transition For Dummies®

Published by: **John Wiley & Sons, Inc.**, 111 River Street, Hoboken, NJ 07030-5774, www.wiley.com

Contents at a Glance

Contents at a Glance

Table of Contents

CHAPTER 15: **Ten Essential Topics to Discuss with Your Healthcare Provider**...................201

CHAPTER 16: **Ten (or So) Trans-Friendly Organizations**...........209

CHAPTER 17: **Ten Ways to Support Transgender and Non-Binary People**...........................215

Introduction

Congratulations on finding this book! Even now, we know that it can be incredibly difficult to get ahold of the resources you need to understand, evaluate, and begin your gender transition journey. Most of our writing team is trans, so we can relate to the excitement and anxiety you may be feeling right now. We're so glad you're here, and we know you'll find some great information in these pages.

Everyone on our team works with and for transgender and non-binary people in the state of New Mexico. Three of us are with the Transgender Resource Center of New Mexico, and one of us is an MD who has treated many trans and non-binary young people and adults. In our combined years of providing services, advocacy, education, and care, we have encountered the same questions over and over.

> » How do I know if I am trans?
>
> » What happens if I take gender-affirming hormones?
>
> » What kinds of surgeries are available for trans people?
>
> » How can I find a supportive healthcare provider?
>
> » How will I handle all of my relationships?

The answers to these questions and more are provided throughout this book, from our own experience and from years of researching answers for our communities.

As you move further into your journey, you'll be faced with complex decisions and situations. Things will be difficult at times, and some folks may experience serious depression and anxiety. Know that you are not alone, and use this resource to find that hand you may need to reach out for when it feels dark.

Transgender and non-binary people have existed throughout human history, even though that's not common knowledge yet. Trans and non-binary people have made huge contributions in many areas of human thought and achievement.

You are part of an unbroken thread of humanity, and you have special gifts to offer the world. Read on for more info and signposts for the road ahead of you.

About This Book

This book was written to compile all the currently known information about gender transition. We wanted to bring together information about medical options, social and legal transition, behavioral health, and personal relationships into one easy-to-access guide.

For the first of many times we note that each person reading this is unique, and your gender transition journey is your own. This book doesn't prescribe a protocol for transition; it's meant to provide you with the information you need to make your own deeply personal decisions about how to proceed and at what pace.

The whole transition process will be easier if you have a good team — healthcare providers you can trust, other trans folks you can talk to, and friends or family who care about and support you. Not everyone is lucky enough to have this support team already in place, so look to this book for some tips and advice about where to begin the search.

Foolish Assumptions

When you're writing a book, it's impossible not to imagine the folks you're talking to on the other side. Imagining you means making some assumptions about you, and here are ours:

» You are transgender or non-binary, or you are a close loved one of someone who is.

» You are interested in taking steps associated with gender transition, or at least want to know what your options are.

» You are looking for scientific and data-based information about the transition process.

» You want to make your own decisions about your transition but would appreciate some information to guide your choices.

» You read and often turn to books like this for guidance.

If this list sounds like it describes you, you've come to the right place. Welcome to *Gender Transition For Dummies!*

Icons Used in This Book

The margins of this book are filled with little cartoons. In the *For Dummies* universe, these are known as *icons*, and they signal certain (we hope) exciting things going on in the accompanying text.

This icon points to practical advice and actionable steps. If you're looking for a clear how-to, this is your go-to marker for helpful suggestions to guide your transition journey.

Whenever you see this icon, know that it highlights something essential — whether it's an important fact or a nugget of wisdom worth keeping in mind. Consider revisiting these worthwhile notes as you move forward.

Gender transition can be a challenging process with risks and pitfalls, whether they're medical, social, or legal. This icon signals areas where extra caution is advised, so that you can navigate these challenges thoughtfully and safely.

Curious about the science behind gender-affirming hormones or the legal details of name changes? This icon introduces in-depth explanations and technical information.

Beyond the Book

In addition to the pages you're reading right now, this book comes with a free, access-anywhere online Cheat Sheet that summarizes some of our key advice at a glance. To access this Cheat Sheet, go to http://www.dummies.com/, and type Gender Transition cheat sheet in the search box.

Where to Go from Here

One option is to read this book from cover to cover to become something of an expert on gender transition. However, you're probably more likely to bounce around from chapter to chapter as you have questions, possibly even returning to this book over months, or even years, as new questions arise and as you reach new inflection points in your personal journey.

If you only want to read about surgeries at this point, you can jump straight to Chapter 9. If you are still really apprehensive and just want to find out more about personal relationships and how they may change during your transition, you can stick with Part 1 for the time being.

It doesn't matter how you use this book. It's here to be both the tour and the guide through the sometimes daunting landscape of gender transition, and we hope it's a great road map for you as you embark on your journey.

1

Getting Familiar with Gender Transition

Chapter **1**

Exploring Gender Transition Elements and Common Questions

I f you're considering transitioning, you've no doubt thought about the many ways that taking this step can change your life. For a lot of people the goal of walking down this path is what some folks today call *gender euphoria* (feelings of satisfaction, confidence, comfort, or even joy that come from being aligned with your gender).

At the same time, challenges and complications may arise for you along the way. You may be someone who came to this book because you are considering this path but really aren't sure yet. That is also absolutely okay.

In the end, nobody but you can know whether this is right for you. Hopefully, though, this book can fill in the gaps in knowledge that you might have, and help provide you with crucial information and perspective to help you with this, sometimes intimidating, decision process.

In this chapter, you find some of the most basic information about what's often called *gender transition* (an array of social, legal, and medical options that some transgender and non-binary people undertake to be more authentically themselves).

You also find definitions of the words *transgender* and *non-binary*, as well as other terms associated with gender and transitioning. (Much more detailed information about social and medical transition is sprinkled throughout the rest of the book, so this chapter is truly an overview.) Finally, we answer some common questions that arise about this topic, including an initial look at finding support and help.

REMEMBER

You may be excited, scared, or confused right now. This book aims to give you more information and provide some pathways to connection and assistance along your journey. Remember that you aren't in this alone, and your transgender or non-binary identity, and your way of relating to it, is valid and valued.

Discovering the Meaning of Transgender and Non-binary

Transgender and non-binary: What do these words mean? Although terminology evolves, the word *transgender* currently refers to anyone whose gender doesn't match up completely with the sex they were designated at birth. *Non-binary* specifically refers to folks who don't feel like either a man or a woman.

As U.S. culture finally recognizes that a child's consistent awareness of their gender typically develops between 2 and 5 years old, it's critical that this awareness doesn't become a hard and fast expectation of ALL transgender and non-binary people. Being transgender or non-binary isn't fully understood by a lot of *cisgender* people (folks whose gender and sex match up 100 percent — in other words, people who aren't transgender), which means that this simple minority characteristic is still stigmatized. Discrimination and violence are strongly correlated with being trans or non-binary, and a lot of people aren't aware of the existence of trans and non-binary people until adulthood, even today! In those circumstances, it's no wonder that many folks don't come to the realization that they're transgender or non-binary, even internally, until later in life. People come out, to themselves and others, in their 20s, 40s, and even their 60s.

Some folks talk about not being able to ask the question "Am I trans?" or "Is there something different about my gender?" until they were much, much older than 5. Another specific time when people tend to start talking about possibly being trans or non-binary, or seeking help from others about gender issues, is at the onset of *natal puberty* (the changes and emergence of secondary sex traits associated with the designated sex at birth).

When the body starts to change in ways that can feel very "wrong" for many trans and non-binary people, those changes can set off an emotional and psychological tailspin. Not everyone experiences this *gender dysphoria* (a thorough definition is found in the section "Answering a Few Common Questions" later in this chapter), and each person's experience is their own. But for a lot of folks, natal puberty is a huge challenge that can worsen all types of behavioral health symptoms, including suicidal thoughts.

TIP

Even trans/non-binary people can struggle when different folks in their lives come out, for a lot of reasons. If you find yourself having a hard time with someone's disclosure about their gender, try to take them at face value. Even if you think they may have something more complex going on, be warm and accepting, and ask open-ended questions about their identity and experience. They thought you were safe enough to confide in, so prove them right!

The bottom line is that right now there's no validating test for someone's gender or for being transgender or non-binary. This means that it can't currently be proved, but it also can't be disproved. Certainly, some folks have questioned their gender and then determined that they weren't trans in the end. But in the initial conversations, it's important not to invalidate a person who needs support (this is great advice for cis folks in your life, too.).

REMEMBER

Don't be hesitant to use any of the words in this section as identity labels — or not! While there are standard definitions for transgender and non-binary, the words people use to describe and define themselves are more like the peel-and-stick name tags folks use at formal events (see Figure 1-1 for an example). You get to write your own label or descriptor on your name tag. Whether a term is generally considered out of date, or may not be used by a majority of folks whose gender is similar to yours, it's up to you how you want to be talked to and talked about. These sticker name tags can be pulled off and exchanged for a new one, if you realize that the one you're wearing isn't working for you anymore.

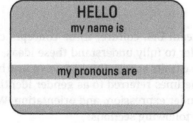

HELLO
my name is

my pronouns are

FIGURE 1-1:
An example of a
self-adhesive
name tag
with pronouns.

Transgender

The word transgender is currently used to mean a person whose designated sex and gender are not the same. It's important to notice that this definition is not binary in nature — meaning that you don't have to feel the opposite of your designated sex to fall under the trans umbrella, just not the same.

When you read about non-binary in the following section, you'll see that non-binary falls under the trans umbrella using these definitions, too. But as we say above, that doesn't mean that a non-binary person has to put on a trans "name tag."

The other critical aspect to stress is that the definition of transgender is not medical in nature. We talk about gender dysphoria more throughout the book, but experiencing gender dysphoria is NOT part of the meaning of transgender. Trans is a shortened version of transgender and is appropriate for anyone to use.

Being transgender or non-binary does not mean that you dress any certain way or adhere to gender norms and stereotypes. It also doesn't indicate anything about your orientation. Trans people fall into every existing category of people, so trans folks can be gay, straight, bisexual, pansexual, asexual, or any other orientation.

Non-binary

Non-binary people have a gender that falls outside the man/woman binary. It's a common misperception that this means that someone who's non-binary is a blend of man and woman. In fact, non-binary describes a wealth of different genders and experiences. Some non-binary people do feel like a mix of man and woman, while others experience no gender at all (sometimes called *agender*).

There are non-binary people who experience their gender as neutral. The term *genderfluid* describes people whose gender shifts and changes over time. This is such a small sampling of ways to be non-binary. If you do not feel like a man, and you also do not feel like a woman, you fall under this non-binary umbrella.

The Four Aspects

For people raised in mainstream U.S. culture, these concepts can feel new and even a little confusing. In order to fully understand these ideas, you must have a grasp of four basic traits. Those traits are sex (broken down into biological sex and designated sex), gender (sometimes referred to as gender identity but not in our trainings or in this book), gender expression, and orientation. We describe these traits more thoroughly in the following sections.

Sex

Sex is a broad term that refers to physiology (how the human body works). It's important to distinguish between biological sex and designated sex, so read on for more information and to find out why.

Biological sex

Biological sex is a complex system formed by five component parts:

>> **Sex chromosomes** are packets of DNA containing the genes that determine someone's sex. XX (female) and XY (male) are the most common examples, but they aren't the only ones humans have.

>> **Sex hormones** are steroid hormones produced by the gonads that cause the development of other secondary sex characteristics. Estrogen and testosterone are the most common examples.

>> **External genitals** (or external genitalia) is the term we use throughout this book to refer to external sex organs. Most commonly, we're talking about the penis/testicles or vulva.

>> **Gonads** is another name for the internal reproductive organs. In humans these are typically testes or ovaries.

>> **Gametes** refers to sex cells (often sperm and ova, or eggs).

Designated sex

Designated sex refers to the sex that was put down on your original birth record. More than 99 percent of the time in the U.S., this designation is made strictly on the basis of external genitals.

The reason you can't interchange the terms biological sex and designated sex is that intersex people exist. *Intersex* currently refers to the estimated 1.7 percent of humans who are born with variations in their biological sex system. In other words, their bodies don't fit the typical definition of male or female. These variations are often very subtle, and there is nothing "wrong" with the bodies of intersex people (just like there is nothing "wrong" with left-handed or red-haired people).

REMEMBER

There are never two kinds of people in the world! For more information about intersex people, check out InterACT Advocates for Intersex Youth (online at https://interactadvocates.org).

Gender

Gender is the term we (and most folks engaged in trans education and advocacy) use to mean the deep, fundamental, internal knowledge that each person has about whether they're a man, a woman, or a non-binary person. This cannot be observed from the outside, which means it can be hidden. If you've been through times in your life when you hid your gender, many people can relate. Hopefully you're now in a place where you can take any steps you want and need to take to live authentically, in alignment with your gender.

REMEMBER

You definitely may have heard gender referred to as "gender identity!" That term is still most often what you will read in protective nondiscrimination laws and policies, and it was the term that even trans folks and trans educators used for many years. As we learn more, the language continues to evolve. When one of our team started teaching about trans people and issues in 2008, trans folks still used the term "preferred gender pronouns." We had gotten so familiar and intimate with that term that we even abbreviated it to "PGPs." After a while though, folks started to realize that we didn't call them "PGPs" when we talked about cisgender folks. And the pronouns of trans folks and cis folks are the same! So now we just say pronouns. Your gender is not the way you "identify." It is (for most folks) a deep, integral, crucial piece of who you are and how you see yourself. For that reason, within the trans and non-binary communities, we typically just use the word gender these days, rather than the outdated and mildly condescending gender identity."

Gender expression

Gender expression is the external aspect of gender, composed of elements such as clothing, hairstyle, jewelry, makeup, speech, gait, gestures, certain preferences, and even many names. This facet of gender is also the most culturally based.

Gender norms and stereotypes vary from one cultural group to another, and they shift over time within a single cultural group. In the U.S., some obvious examples of gender norms shifting over time include women having access to the same professions men work in, as well as men choosing to be stay-at-home dads. Kilts and skirts are terrific examples of how the same item can be classified as masculine or feminine depending on the cultural group you're raised in. After all, a piece of fabric that wraps around your waist can't be masculine or feminine on its own. These expectations and definitions that many people are taught from the first moments of their lives can change throughout your lifetime.

Orientation

Orientation refers to a person's romantic, physical, emotional, and/or sexual attraction — or lack of attraction — to other people. Some of the relative terms used to describe orientation are *straight* (opposite-gender attraction), *gay* (same-gender attraction), *bisexual* (attraction to two or more genders), *pansexual* (individualized attraction to any gender), and *asexual* (lack of sexual attraction to others). Asexual, sometimes called "ace," refers to a wide range of experiences around sex. Being asexual certainly doesn't mean that you don't like people. It may not even mean that you don't engage in sex. Some asexual folks enjoy having sex, but others may not feel that way. These attitudes can be referred to as sex positive, sex neutral, or sex negative asexual. Asexual also does not specify a person's experience, or interest in, romantic attraction. One person could be panromantic and asexual, for example. And guess what? Straight, gay, bi, pansexual and asexual aren't the only options. There is so much more to learn when it comes to orientation and attraction.

REMEMBER

Each of the four attributes described in the preceding sections is separate and distinct from the others. Trans and non-binary people are defined by having a sex and gender that don't match. Likewise, someone's gender expression may not be linked with their internal gender. There's actually no way to "look" non-binary. And think of people like RuPaul, a cisgender man who elaborately dresses like a woman, but not to show that he feels like a woman internally. The acronym LGBT (which stands for lesbian, gay, bisexual, and transgender) may make it sound like orientation and gender are linked, but even those pieces are separate. Just like a cisgender person, a trans person can be gay, straight, bi, or any other orientation.

A HISTORICAL PERSPECTIVE OF TRANSGENDER AND NON-BINARY PEOPLE

One of the most important things to remember is that transgender and non-binary people are not new. Cultures throughout human history have recognized more than two defined gender categories — some acknowledge as many as seven! Many languages contain words and categories for transgender and non-binary people, such as the Polynesian fa'afafine. Transgender and non-binary individuals have existed throughout history, way before the advent of modern medical transition. The Public Universal Friend and Albert Cashier (you can search Wikipedia for more info about both) are just two examples. Joe Stevens, a very talented trans musician, actually co-wrote a musical about Albert. It's called *The Civility of Albert Cashier*, and you can learn more about it and Joe at the website https://www.albertcashiermusical.com/.

This history is often associated with ancient and/or Indigenous cultures, and some of those societies definitely did recognize multiple gender categories. But even in the

(continued)

(continued)

modern era, you can find examples of gender variance worldwide. Hijras in India and Muxe in Mexico are good examples. Even in the United States, the first group that could be seen as a transgender advocacy group came about in New York City in 1895! It was called the Cercle Hermaphroditos.

Even though the concept feels new in a lot of places, including the U.S., understanding that transgender and non-binary people have always existed helps ground them in human history and establishes that trans people represent a normal human variation, or minority characteristic. Because a small percentage of humans are born trans or non-binary, being trans/non-binary is actually similar to being left-handed or having red hair — both great examples of minority traits.

Lefties and redheads also have a well-documented history of being misunderstood, looked down on, and persecuted, but both groups are fairly well integrated into U.S. culture at this point. In fact, it's not difficult to find left-handed notebooks, can openers, guitars, rifles, and even golf clubs! In 1971, an article in the *Florence (AL) Times — Tri-Cities Daily* entitled "New Day Dawns for Southpaws" included the quote "Left-handers — not to be confused with leftists — are becoming increasingly accepted and enabled to take their right (or left) place in the world." This provides hope that transgender and non-binary people will someday be treated with the same casual acceptance that society displays toward left-handed people today.

Exploring the Changes Involved in Gender Transition

The gender transition steps and options we outline in this book may be some of the best things you ever do for yourself; still, many people have a significant fear of change and the unknown. A little information can go a long way in easing that anxiety, and this book has a lot of information.

It's important to realize going into this journey that each step you take can be something that changes your body, your confidence, your relationships, your work or school life, and your family. Of course, this can be true about any decisions you make for yourself throughout your life. The choice to have children, be in committed romantic relationships, take or leave a job, or move to a new place can also have big ramifications. We want you to know that this may not be completely smooth sailing, but that's true about life in general!

Taking hormones or having surgery will result in major changes to your body and the way you experience it. We detail the masculinizing and feminizing effects of hormones in Chapter 8, but in general, hormones will cause huge shifts in your feelings and in various aspects of your body. If you opt for what is considered a full masculinizing or feminizing dose of hormones, you'll actually restart puberty. For some transgender and non-binary people who begin this process later in life, this can mean going through full puberty twice. They will experience many of the changes and challenges related to puberty, including

>> Physical

>> Developmental

>> Cognitive

>> Psychological

When you're aware of this, and get the support you need, it's a lot easier to get through it. You may even be the person who sometimes reassures your loved ones that puberty is a process, and that it eventually comes to an end.

Socially and professionally, things can unfold in a lot of different ways. For some people who transition very little changes in the reality of their day-to-day lives. Some trans or non-binary people stay in the relationships they're in when they begin the process, and work for employers who are supportive and affirming. For some people, their children, young or older, are their biggest cheerleaders. So, try not to assume that everything will only be negative once you begin showing up as the person you're meant to be.

However, it's misleading to suggest that people don't ever run into challenges, large and small, as a result of charting their course through these waters. Some people have family members, partners, or children who don't accept them as they start to tell the truth about who they are. Some folks lose their jobs, and others have a hard time finding new employment after embarking on transition-related changes. We address many of these challenges, as well as the ways some people have managed them, in Chapters 3 and 12.

Despite the potential issues, the data indicates that people who take steps to transition are quite satisfied. Figure 1-2 shows the data from the 2022 U.S. Transgender Survey on how many trans and non-binary people report high levels of satisfaction with the steps they took to transition.

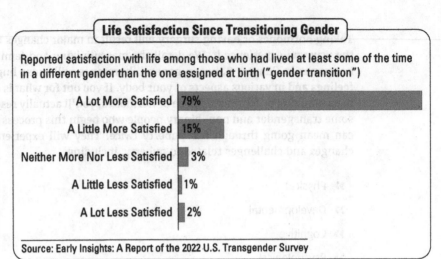

FIGURE 1-2:
A table from the 2022 U.S. Transgender Survey addressing satisfaction levels with gender transition.

Understanding the Life Implications of Transitioning

Because each trans and non-binary person is on an individual path, we can't provide a standard recipe or certain order for how to proceed with your transition. That also means we can't fully predict what the implications of the steps you take will be. The one thing you can be sure of, though, is that things will definitely be different in many ways once you start making changes like the ones we explore in this book.

Many areas of your life can be impacted when you decide to be your authentic self and move toward your genuine presentation of who you are and/or the creation of a body that's the right home for you. Although many people don't experience these things, and others don't report them as negatives, some of the fundamental issues people share about transition that can be challenging include

>> Body changes that are less desirable, such as decreased strength for people taking estrogen, and pattern baldness or even increased difficulty freely crying for some people on testosterone

>> Unwanted social attention in public

>> Fear of seeking out medical care

» Difficulty at work or obtaining employment

» Dating challenges

» Discrimination

» Fears about blending in or "passing"

» Difficulty navigating existing romantic and family relationships

» Unfamiliar gender stereotypes (for example, a trans man who hasn't been perceived as a man in the past may face aggressive behavior from other men, such as being challenged to a fight)

On the other hand, transgender and non-binary people have cited the following things as the upside of transitioning:

» Confidence, happiness, and peace of mind

» Freedom to make other big decisions that will improve their lives

» Easing of some behavioral health symptoms

» Less or no substance misuse

» An end to suicidal thoughts

» More involvement in their medical care and well-being

» Dreams and hopes for the future

REMEMBER

The real-world consequences of transitioning can sound intimidating, but don't let doubt or anxiety hold you back from checking out the options you believe are right for you. As Figure 1-2 demonstrates, the majority of trans and non-binary people who take these steps report lifelong satisfaction with them. Plus, very few transition-related changes are truly irreversible. It's okay to explore!

Answering a Few Common Questions

You may be wondering about some transition-related issues, or you may have friends or family who are curious about these topics. The following sections provide answers to a handful of questions some folks may have.

Does everyone have gender dysphoria?

The American Psychiatric Association's (APA) *Diagnostic and Statistical Manual of Mental Disorders*, 5th Edition (*DSM-5*), currently defines *gender dysphoria* as

A marked incongruence between one's experienced/expressed gender and assigned gender, of at least six months' duration, as manifested by at least two or more of the following:

>> A marked incongruence between one's experienced/expressed gender and primary and/or secondary sex characteristics (or in young adolescents, the anticipated secondary sex characteristics)

>> A strong desire to be rid of one's primary and/or secondary sex characteristics because of a marked incongruence with one's experienced/expressed gender (or in young adolescents, a desire to prevent the development of the antici-pated secondary sex characteristics)

>> A strong desire for the primary and/or secondary sex characteristics of the other gender

>> A strong desire to be of the other gender (or some alternative gender different from one's assigned gender)

>> A strong desire to be treated as the other gender (or some alternative gender different from one's assigned gender)

>> A strong conviction that one has the typical feelings and reactions of the other gender (or some alternative gender different from one's assigned gender)

The condition is associated with clinically significant distress or impairment in social, occupational, or other important areas of functioning.

WARNING

Another book can be written (and probably has been!) about the complex and troubling history of the *DSM-5*. One brief example is that the *DSM* classified being gay as a "mental disorder" from its first edition in 1952 up to the seventh printing of the second edition in 1974.

While gender dysphoria helps many trans and non-binary people organize and understand their experiences and serves as the needed justification for coverage of gender-affirming treatment by insurance carriers, who almost all pay for this treatment now, the APA's current definition of the term must be taken with a grain of salt given the DSM's past.

Does every trans person experience gender dysphoria? The answer is no! But folks can't be blamed for thinking that gender dysphoria is essential to being transgender or non-binary. Most media coverage and representation has focused on trans people who both experience gender dysphoria and undergo medical treatment for it.

REMEMBER

The definition of being transgender is that your internal gender — that internal knowing about being a man, a woman, or a non-binary person — doesn't completely match the sex you were designated at birth (in other words, the sex that was recorded on your first birth certificate). It's absolutely possible to know that about yourself and not simultaneously harbor angry or hateful feelings toward your body. As always, remember that each transgender and non-binary person is an individual, and your experience is your own.

What about cisgender people? Since the current definition of gender dysphoria specifically references the incongruence, or disconnect, between designated sex and gender, cisgender folks, by definition, cannot experience gender dysphoria. They certainly can, and sometimes do, feel deep and debilitating insecurities about their gender, their body, and their gender presentation.

Cisgender women who undergo mastectomies for breast cancer, or who have naturally thinning hair or bald patches, can face unsolicited feedback from strangers about their femininity and appeal. Cisgender men who have wide hips or aren't able to grow a thick, full beard may face the same criticism, or may just suffer internally with feelings of inadequacy about their masculinity. In fact, if you think about it, many, if not most, cosmetic surgeries can be considered gender-affirming surgeries. They often represent a person's efforts to obtain the stereotypical ideal of how a man or woman is supposed to appear.

TIP

The prefix "cis" is a Latin prefix meaning "lined up on the same side." Trans is the natural opposite in Latin, meaning "crossing over." When you look at these prefixes, much like "pre" and "post," you can see that they belong together in a set. A cis person has a gender and sex that line up, or match, while trans and non-binary folks have crossing over of some kind between those two things. Cisgender is not in any way a hateful or derogatory term, no matter what you hear. It is really most like the word *right-handed*, in other words, a neutral word for the dominant, majority group.

How do I know if I'm transgender?

If you're asking yourself this question, you should know that you're not alone. Many people before you have taken this same interior journey. There's nothing wrong with you, and no matter what the answer turns out to be, this questioning process is a great opportunity to understand more deeply who you are.

In short, if you fit the definition of transgender — your gender is different from the sex you were designated at birth — then you are trans. This is definitely not meant to be a glib answer, because being transgender contains a world of nuance and variations.

For example, many people can feel like a man or a woman and still be uncomfortable with or resent the gender norms and stereotypes they face in that gender. Enjoying the clothes, activities, or stereotypical interests of one gender or another doesn't make you that gender. Every tomboy isn't a transgender boy, and many drag queens are cisgender gay men who don't feel deeply that they're women internally. Some male pop stars have incorporated so-called women's clothing into their stage or street looks, dating back to the 1960s. Conversely, you can be a transgender man and enjoy performing as a drag queen.

REMEMBER

Deep internal knowledge of being a man, woman, or non-binary person doesn't obligate you to adhere to the norms and expectations your culture associates with that group. To put it another way, gender expression isn't gender.

Many transgender and non-binary adults will tell you that sometime between the ages of 2 and 5, they knew their gender, and that their knowledge was unexpected and sometimes unwanted by their parents and others. Although some people find that astonishing, it's the common experience of kids across the board. The American Academy of Pediatrics (AAP) has affirmed that awareness of gender is a typical part of a child's development. The AAP's parenting website, Healthy Children.org, repeatedly reinforces that gender identity typically develops in the following stages:

>> **Around age 2:** Children become conscious of the physical differences between boys and girls.

>> **Before their 3rd birthday:** Most children can easily label themselves as either a boy or a girl.

>> **By age 4:** Most children have a stable sense of their gender identity.

During this same time of life, children learn gender role behavior — that is, how to do "things that boys do" or "things that girls do." However, cross-gender preferences and play are a normal part of gender development and exploration regardless of a child's future gender identity (see "The Power of Play: How Fun and Games Help Children Thrive" on HealthyChildren.org).

The point is that all children tend to develop a clearer view of themselves and their gender over time. Research suggests that children who assert a gender-diverse identity at any point in childhood know their gender as clearly and consistently as their developmentally matched peers and benefit from the same level of support, love, and social acceptance (https://www.healthychildren.org/English/ages-stages/gradeschool/Pages/Gender-Identity-and-Gender-Confusion-In-Children.aspx).

And according to the American Psychological Association's paper "Gender Diversity and Transgender Identity in Children" (https://www.apadivisions.org/division-44/resources/advocacy/transgender-children.pdf):

Transgender children typically consistently, persistently, and insistently express a cross-gender identity and feel that their gender is different from their assigned sex. They may begin talking about their gender as soon as they begin to speak and some may express dissatisfaction with their genitals. Transgender children are more likely to experience gender dysphoria (i.e., discomfort related to their bodies not matching their internal sense of gender) than gender diverse children, although some transgender children are comfortable with their bodies. Transgender children may state that they are really the other gender, or that someone (e.g., the doctor or a religious authority) made a mistake in their gender assignment.

Whether you knew this about yourself from a very young age or you're just starting to investigate your gender, don't be deterred. Neither route makes you more trans than someone else.

Some strategies you can use to explore questions about your gender include the following:

>> **Meet transgender and non-binary folks and talk to them about their experiences.** Yours don't have to be identical, but sharing can help you see possible patterns of common experiences.

>> **Join an online or in-person support group.** There may already be some trans/non-binary groups meeting in your area, but if not there are some online for youth, adults, and family members.

>> **Talk to a safe and supportive therapist or counselor.** This can be one of the most important things you do for yourself. Trans and non-binary people experience negative outcomes throughout our lives, and therapy, especially therapy that focuses on trauma, can be really transformational, beyond just the transition process. (see Chapter 13 for more in-depth information).

>> **Experiment with changing elements of your gender expression as safely as you can.** Sometimes playing around with your gender expression elicits a strong emotional reaction that can give you more information.

>> **Read books and articles on the subject.** You can find helpful information in books such as *The Gender Quest Workbook* (https://www.newharbinger.com/9781626252974/the-gender-quest-workbook/).

Is someone I love transgender?

This question can be scary, even if you are trans or non-binary yourself. A lot of parents feel anxious and protective of their kids, and often experience initial worry and fear about their child having a minority trait that may put them in harm's way. For kids asking this question about a parent, it can seem as if everything will change if it turns out to be true.

REMEMBER

If you're asking this question about someone in your life, try not to worry. Your loved one is absolutely the person you know them to be, whether they're trans or not. And they need your support for the journey ahead if they are.

Finding Help and Support for Navigating Gender Transition

You can get much more information about seeking out supportive relationships, finding a therapist, and taking advantage of online resources in Chapters 3 and 12, so our most important point in this section is to encourage you to realize that you need help and support. Mainstream U.S. culture emphasizes self-sufficiency, individualism, and stoicism (not showing emotions). But human beings are built for connection and community.

The groundbreaking 2023 report "Our Epidemic of Loneliness and Isolation: The U.S. Surgeon General's Advisory on the Healing Effects of Social Connection and Community" (https://www.hhs.gov/sites/default/files/surgeon-general-social-connection-advisory.pdf) states the following:

> The lack of social connection poses a significant risk for individual health and longevity. Loneliness and social isolation increase the risk for premature death by 26% and 29% respectively.

> More broadly, lacking social connection can increase the risk for premature death as much as smoking up to 15 cigarettes a day. In addition, poor or insufficient social connection is associated with increased risk of disease, including a 29% increased risk of heart disease and a 32% increased risk of stroke. Furthermore, it is associated with increased risk for anxiety, depression, and dementia. Additionally, the lack of social connection may increase susceptibility to viruses and respiratory illness.

Some tried-and-true ideas for trying to forge connections include

>> **Be yourself.** That's what this book is all about. And as you figure out who you are and what you need to feel authentic, other people will notice too.

>> **Be present.** In today's technological and fast-paced world this can be a big challenge. Putting aside your devices, even for 5 minutes, and being present with others is one of the main ways to connect.

>> **Be forgiving of yourself.** A lot of folks talk to themselves in ways that they would never speak to someone else. Everyone deserves a little slack for being a human who sometimes makes mistakes. That includes you.

>> **Be mindful that vulnerability is power.** Author Brené Brown once said in an interview, "There is no courage without vulnerability. Vulnerability is not weakness. It's the ability to show up and be seen. It's the ability to be brave when you cannot control the outcome."

TIP

There isn't just one way, or right way, to seek support. Each person is different and has different needs. You don't have to go through this experience alone, though. Whether you seek out professional help, new friends, or a support group, find your team. You may feel much more comfortable seeking help online than in person. Pay attention to your boundaries and needs, but try not to isolate yourself.

The transition process is exciting and challenging, but don't forget that many people have walked this road before you in their own way.

Chapter 2

Looking More Closely at Gender Transition

You hear it many times from us throughout this book: There are as many different transitions as there are transgender and non-binary people. What works great for someone else may not be right for you, and vice versa. It's a lot to consider, but remember that you're the expert on you. In the end you have to inhabit the choices you make along your journey, so the most important person to clear them with is yourself.

In this chapter, we help you survey the broad landscape of gender transition. Starting with the social side of transition, you find information about the changes that may come, and begin to think about and set your personal goals for your transition process.

This chapter also illuminates the basics of medical transition. You uncover the overall picture of what's available and how to make decisions about what's right for you.

REMEMBER

Transitioning is complicated stuff, and you don't have to have all the answers at this point. This book aims to be a guide that lays out a lot of information to help you puzzle your way through everything in the transition process.

Examining Social Transition

The phrase *social transition* refers to any transition-related steps that don't fall into the medical realm. Part 2 of this book is all about social transition, so in this chapter we just provide a basic overview. Some common elements of social transition are

>> **Coming out:** For many people, coming out is one of the first and most significant steps in social transition. This can mean disclosing your gender to family, friends, colleagues, or the wider community. Coming out isn't a single event but an ongoing process of sharing your truth with others in various contexts. It can be empowering, but also challenging, as you navigate others' reactions and establish boundaries.

>> **Changing your clothes:** Clothing is a powerful form of self-expression, and changing how you dress can be an important part of your social transition. This may involve adopting clothing styles that are more traditionally masculine, feminine, or gender-neutral. Clothing choices can impact how you're perceived by others and contribute to your sense of authenticity.

>> **Shifting your mannerisms, including the way you walk:** Mannerisms, such as the way you move, gesture, or even speak, are often tied to gender stereotypes. When you're undergoing a social transition, you may try adjusting your mannerisms. This may involve altering how you walk, carry yourself, or interact with others — small but significant changes that can contribute to a more comfortable and authentic presentation of yourself.

>> **Adjusting your hairstyle:** Hair is another key element in gender expression. You may choose to change your hairstyle — cutting your hair short, growing it out, or choosing a new style altogether — as part of your social transition. The way you wear your hair can have a strong impact on how you feel and how others perceive your gender.

>> **Trying out makeup:** Experimenting with makeup can be a fun and important step for some folks. This may include discovering new makeup techniques, experimenting with different looks, or simply incorporating makeup into your daily routine as a way to be more confident and, sometimes, more visible in your authentic gender.

>> **Tucking, binding, and using prostheses:** As part of your social transition, you may take specific steps to alter your body's shape under your clothing. *Tucking* (minimizing the appearance of a penis or "bulge"), *binding* (flattening the chest with compression), and using *prostheses* (such as breast forms or a prosthetic penis, usually called a packer) are common practices you can use to feel more comfortable in your body or to match your gender with your gender

presentation. These practices are often temporary and can be a way to create a more assured presentation while navigating social spaces.

>> **Changing your name/pronouns:** One of the most significant and public aspects of social transition can be changing your name and pronouns. This may involve informing family, friends, coworkers, and the broader community of your new name and pronouns. Although some people choose to formally change their name through legal processes, others may opt for informal changes, especially if they aren't ready or able to go through legal channels. You'll be amazed how good it feels to have the right name and pronouns coming out of the mouths of folks around you!

>> **Using a new bathroom:** One of the most immediate and practical aspects of social transition is choosing to use the bathroom that aligns with your gender. This can be a highly sensitive issue, because some people face resistance or discrimination in public spaces. Navigating bathroom use may be a significant challenge, particularly if you're gender-nonconforming or in the early stages of your transition.

>> **Updating your legal documents and IDs:** Although this step involves legal processes, it's often part of the broader social transition. Updating documents like driver's licenses, Social Security records, and other forms of identification to reflect your gender can be a critical part of your transition. Having legal documents that reflect your true identity can help you move through the world with less friction and fewer instances of *misgendering* (being identified as the wrong gender).

Social transition is powerful. A 2023 study published by the National Library of Medicine reported that early social transition by transgender minors "had positive and immediate benefits on child development as well as in the reduction of anxiety. There was a general improvement in mood, self-esteem, and social and family relationships." This information was collected from immediate family members in a focus group setting. And even though you may not be a youth (like this study concentrated on), we have helped and observed hundreds, maybe even thousands, of trans and non-binary adults of all ages along their transition journeys and have seen people experience the gender euphoria of social transition with our own eyes.

Setting objectives for your transition

Being on your own path can be really freeing, because it means you're the person who gets to decide what you want and need to fully realize your gender and become the person you know you're supposed to be. But it can also be a little bit intimidating. Even though other folks have been brave enough to come out and openly walk their path, nobody can truly set the example for your transition. So, it's good to spend some time thinking about all the available options and setting some goals for yourself.

This book is a great guide to help you investigate the different elements that can be part of a gender transition. You can use it and other resources to do some research and spend time mentally trying on some of your options. Finding social support and connecting with other trans or non-binary people is also a great idea at this time (see Chapter 12 for more on reaching out to others for support). You may already feel pretty sure about what you need to do, but if you're still figuring it out, then talking to folks who've taken the steps you're interested in can give you much more information about what's involved in transition and the possible outcomes you can expect.

Once you have the information you need, it's time to lay it all out and try to create your personal road map. For most people transition isn't a strict linear process, and some steps will most likely overlap with others. But in general, a lot of people venture into the process by coming out to others first, and then altering their appearance and trying out new names and pronouns before legally changing their name or updating their identity documents.

REMEMBER

You may feel a sense of urgency and want to move as quickly as you can, or you may prefer to be very deliberate and take your time to adjust to each new step — and to allow others to adjust too. Again, there's no standard transition process, so try to trust your gut. And remember that support from real people is invaluable. Whether you turn to a friend, family member, support group, or therapist, talking over your decisions with someone else, and not keeping everything inside, can really help you put things in perspective.

Understanding the social changes that may come

You may have spent a lot of time dreaming of the transition you're about to undertake. Depending on how long you've been aware that you're trans or non-binary, and how long you've known that gender transition is available, your transition may be many years in the making. Some people in your life may not be at all surprised when you come out, because they expected it all along. For others, though, it may feel more sudden. Either way, your transition can bring up a lot of feelings for some folks, including grief and uncertainty about how it changes things for them. This can be hard to deal with, when you are possibly feeling excited and vulnerable about sharing yourself with the world. Make sure you get support for whatever processes the folks around you go through, especially if the beginning is bumpy.

If the people around you do struggle with what's happening, that doesn't mean they reject you or don't love you. Even feelings of grief are part of an overall emotional process. Although some trans and non-binary people are rejected by friends and family members when they come out, others simply have people in their lives who need time and space to work through their "stuff."

It can be tempting to help them do this, but it's much better to let them find another outlet for their feelings instead. Turning to an experienced therapist or a support group for family members is a great option, but even talking to other trusted confidants is better than asking you to work things through with them. If you can, try to be patient and know that they really do care for you.

You may also notice changes in how people you don't know well, or at all, interact with you after you begin to transition. If you don't experience *gender dysphoria* (distress or discomfort because your gender and assigned sex don't match) or don't make any physical or legal changes, you may find that the treatment you receive from others after you come out is frustrating.

You know yourself to be the gender you truly are, and you may have told important people in your life, but people you meet from day to day won't be able to see this or know it. This can be really discouraging and cause you to experience *social dysphoria* (discomfort triggered by interactions with people who misgender you).

Some trans people who transition experience discrimination and threats from others. This is most common for trans women and trans feminine people, and for non-binary and trans masculine people who are *visibly transgender* (meaning that people often assume they're trans simply from observing them). People in this category bear much of the brunt of the discrimination and violence aimed at trans and non-binary folks. We dive into more detail about these experiences in Chapter 3.

Other trans and non-binary people actually gain unearned social privilege (advantages that are only available to certain people based on characteristics they have) from the changes they make. We don't know of anyone who transitioned in order to increase their social or cultural privilege, but for some trans folks, it's inevitable.

This is especially true for white trans masculine people who take testosterone and assimilate, or blend in. For trans men of color, the reality is more nuanced, or subtle. Traveling a path from being perceived as a Black woman to being perceived as a Black man in the United States is definitely not a simple gain in privilege. And for folks on the femme side, it's almost always a reduction in social privilege, too.

REMEMBER

Regardless of your individual characteristics or the course of your personal transition, you'll definitely find that people react differently to you before and after. How that looks and feels for you will depend on all of your intersecting identity traits (such as your race, age, sexuality, nationality, disability, neurodivergence, gender, and appearance) and the steps you take (or don't take) on your gender journey.

Finally, the most unexpected sphere of change brought on by transition is often internal. You may not be thinking about all the different feelings you'll have as part of this process, and all the ways your self-image will change. You may struggle with the new reality of other people's reactions, whether they're positive or negative.

You may actually have some grief of your own, for the many different elements of the gender or gender role you're leaving behind. Chapter 12 offers some suggestions about how to find support during this time.

Delving into Medical Transition: Looking at Your Options

The details of medical transition are described in Part 3, but an overview is important here. Medical transition is almost always the first thing people think of when they hear the word *transition,* or the phrase *gender transition.* The social and legal elements of transition can be powerful for many trans people; a legal name change is life-altering. But in the popular imagination, and maybe in your mind, too, medical transition looms large as a central piece of being trans.

TIP

For that reason, it can't be overstated that medical steps are *not* a prerequisite for being transgender or non-binary. You may feel a lot of pressure to display your gender externally in ways that other people understand and relate to, but you are the person who has to live with your gender and your gender expression.

Being trans offers you a great chance to accept and love yourself, and figure out who you are to the best of your ability!

The highlights of medical transition are

>> Gender-affirming primary care

>> Hair removal

>> Hormone therapy

>> Fertility and *cryopreservation* (freezing and storage) of genetic tissue

>> Voice modification

>> Surgeries (which may be different than you think — check out Chapter 9)

Deciding on treatment, therapy, and ongoing care

What types of transition-related medical care you want and need is probably one of the most common, and urgent, decisions that trans and non-binary people must make. It feels fraught to have to select medical treatments from all the options that will change your life dramatically. A few of these treatments are considered irreversible, which further complicates your choices.

TIP

Remember, it's a great idea to seek out trusted people you can brainstorm and consult with. Others can't make your decisions for you, but a lot of people process tough choices better when they can talk about them out loud and get meaningful feedback from someone they trust. A mental health therapist may be a good option, but you may prefer a trans support group or just a smart, caring friend or family member.

Attempting to forecast the changes medical transition brings — what they mean, how they'll feel, and how you'll react to them — can be challenging, but it's worth a try. This requires you to investigate the treatment options you're curious about. Part 3 of this book provides a lot of information, but you may want to do some further digging, such as trying to find first-person accounts from folks who've had a procedure or treatment you're considering.

For some trans women and trans feminine people, a *vaginoplasty* (surgical construction of a vagina) is a vital step on their gender transition path, and at the same time, the commitment to daily *dilation* (using a medical dilator — similar to a dildo — to keep the surgically created vaginal canal from closing up) can seem like a big burden.

Doing research doesn't mean that what you hear or read will change your mind. It just means that you'll have all the necessary information as you begin to take steps that sometimes bring bigger changes than you expected.

Other factors in your decision-making may include whether you have health insurance, what your insurance covers, whether you have any health issues that may interact with your treatments, and whether you have access to nearby health-care providers and treatments. In addition, worries and fears about how other people are going to react can sometimes influence transition care decisions.

All these factors, along with your initial decisions, can change over time. Right now, you may feel like you need surgery but no hormones (or some other combination of treatments). In time, even over several years, you may come to understand that taking hormones is an important step in your journey.

Everyone changes, in many ways, throughout their life, so of course it's true that trans and non-binary people change. Accept that change happens in many areas of your life, not just in your gender and gender transition — and that's okay!

Understanding the physical changes you face

In terms of physical changes, the shifts that take place during medical transition depend on your body and the treatments you opt for. It's very hard to predict how things will unfold, but we can give you a general idea about what to expect.

Hormones cause a wide array of changes, many of which you can read about in Chapter 8. Folks report emotional, physical, psychological, and developmental shifts. If you decide to undergo hormone therapy at what's considered the typical doses, you'll initiate a second puberty.

This doesn't have to be a huge deal, but it will involve some mood swings and developmental shifts in your thinking and emotions.

REMEMBER

Puberty usually lasts about four years, so don't be surprised if you go through physical and emotional changes and unexpected responses for a similar length of time. You really will come out the other side! Nobody's puberty has lasted forever.

Surgery is a big step, no matter what type you have. Even surgeries unrelated to being trans or non-binary are major life events that require a lot of healing and can be disruptive to your routine. So, surgeries that bring your body into alignment with your gender may be incredibly exciting and fulfilling, but they may also arouse complicated feelings and pose some logistical challenges for you.

Don't be shocked if your feelings are all over the place. Medical transition brings relief and gender euphoria for a lot of people. Feeling insecure, struggling with internalized transphobia, having anxiety about dating and job hunting, and worrying about the decisions you're making are also natural responses and don't mean that anything is wrong with you.

Talking about your feelings and working through them is part of the transition process for a lot of transgender and non-binary people. Your emotions can be intense during this time, but those feelings often pass and don't cause most people to truly doubt their transition goals or steps, or to want to change anything about what they've done.

TECHNICAL STUFF

The Early Insights Report from the 2022 U.S. Transgender Survey shows that satisfaction rates (either "a lot more satisfied" or "a little more satisfied") were 94 percent or higher for the following questions:

>> Reported satisfaction with life for people who've lived at least some of the time in a different gender than the one they were assigned at birth — that is, they've undergone some gender transition. (See Figure 2-1).

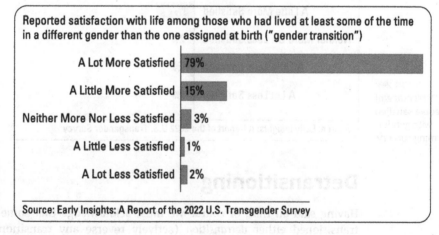

Reported satisfaction with life among those who had lived at least some of the time in a different gender than the one assigned at birth ("gender transition")

A Lot More Satisfied	79%
A Little More Satisfied	15%
Neither More Nor Less Satisfied	3%
A Little Less Satisfied	1%
A Lot Less Satisfied	2%

Source: Early Insights: A Report of the 2022 U.S. Transgender Survey

FIGURE 2-1: Percentage of people satisfied with gender transition.

>> Level of satisfaction with life since receiving hormone treatment for gender identity/transition (See Figure 2-2).

>> Level of satisfaction with life since receiving surgery for gender identity/transition (See Figure 2-3.)

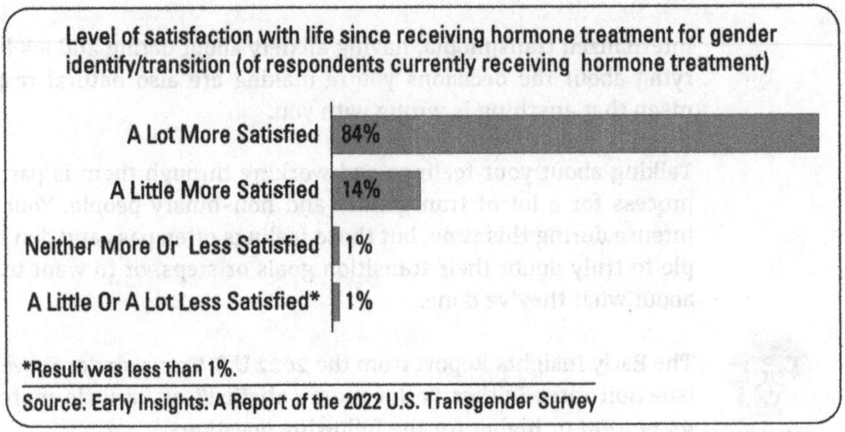

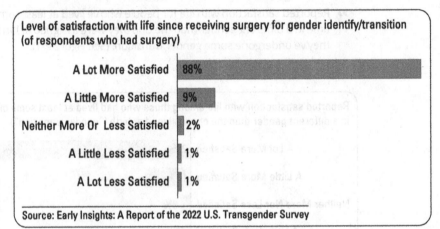

FIGURE 2-2: Percentage of people satisfied with hormone use for gender transition.

FIGURE 2-3: Percentage of people satisfied with gender-affirming surgery.

Detransitioning

Having said all that, of course we must acknowledge that some people who've transitioned either *detransition* (actively reverse any transition steps they've taken) or *desist* (stop wherever they are and forgo any further transition steps). The data shows that about 1 percent of folks regret having gender-affirming surgeries. Some people temporarily detransition but eventually go back to their true gender.

A study from the Fenway Institute published in *LGBT Health* found that 13.1 percent of the transgender people surveyed had detransitioned at some point, but

82.5 percent of them cited at least one external factor for their decision, such as pressure from family, a non-affirming environment, or increased vulnerability to violence, including sexual assault.

It seems clear that the number of people who detransition is pretty low, and their reasons are complex and often about something other than regret over gender-affirming treatment.

In fact, one study showed that a significant number of people who detransition uncovered their non-binary identity while they were transitioning to a binary gender, which changed their track regarding medical transition. Another study outlined some of the most common reasons people detransition:

>> Pressure from a parent (36%)

>> Transitioning was too hard (33%)

>> Too much harassment or discrimination (31%)

>> Trouble getting a job (29%)

REMEMBER

Almost all medical treatments have a documented percentage of patient regret. Different studies report different rates, but the reported rate of regret for back surgery ranges from 8 percent to 22 percent. That's much higher than any regret for gender-related surgeries.

Chapter **3**

Planning for and Adapting with Gender Transition

I n Chapter 2, we review the basic elements of social and medical transition, and some of the shifts that can take place as a result of your transition. Now, it's time for a more in-depth look at how all this affects the different relationships in your life.

In this chapter, you plunge into the many changes that will happen as a result of your gender transition. In addition to finding out about legal steps you must take and getting clarity on how your sexuality may develop and change, you uncover information about searching for a supportive community and choosing a new name that represents your true self.

You may be thinking, "I'm not sure there are any supportive people where I live!" But don't despair. Although it's not the same, you can definitely find real people online who are out there waiting to welcome you. And you may be surprised at the people around you, too. Transgender and non-binary people exist everywhere in the world, and that means their parents, siblings, kids, friends, and partners are everywhere, too.

REMEMBER

Of course, you'll also come across people who aren't supportive or who may even openly oppose and reject you. This is part of the current cultural reality, which we also touch on in this chapter.

Establishing a Supportive Community

How do you start to create a caring, accepting community for yourself? This can feel like a lot to grapple with alongside all the other decisions you're making right now. Figuring out your personal gender transition, and then engaging in the steps you decide to take, is one of the biggest projects you'll undertake in your life.

It takes up a lot of time, sometimes a great deal of money, and a huge amount of mental and emotional energy. Many people worry whether they are making the "right" decisions, and are legitimately afraid of losing important relationships in their life because of the path they're now pursuing.

Even if you transition later in life, you'll very likely find yourself having to think deeply about who you are, what you want, and how you want to live your life. The necessity of making sure you have strong, connected relationships may feel like one more thing you aren't sure you have the energy for.

But the investment you make in building and strengthening your community will reward you with rich dividends throughout your transition and beyond.

Looking for connections locally and online

In an ideal world, you'll have some friends before you begin the process who love and respect you and stick with you during and after your transition. When you have even a couple of reliable, loving people in your life who hang in there for the long term (whether you're trans/non-binary or not), that's a great gift that will absolutely be a big help in getting through everything.

But for some people who are transitioning, this may not be the case. You may have struggled to make good friends before you came out, or you may be one of the many people in the transgender communities who have valued relationships fall away when you begin to tell the truth about who you are.

REMEMBER

Nothing can immediately take away the pain of being rejected by other people. This is true when you're a kid trying to make friends, or when you try out for a part in a play and don't get it. For trans and non-binary people, rejection is complicated by the fact that you're finally being open and honest about who you really know yourself to be. Being rejected in the face of that type of vulnerability is especially hurtful.

Try to remember that it's absolutely not about you. If someone pulls away only because you reveal that you're transgender or non-binary, their behavior is a reflection on their character, not yours. The passage of time eases the sting of rejection for a lot of people. Also, turning your attention to forging new connections is the surest way to move forward and heal from abandonment.

YOU CAN FIND FRIENDS AND ALLIES ANYWHERE

The Transgender Resource Center of New Mexico (TGRCNM) has delivered more than 4,000 transgender cultural fluency trainings to doctors, nurses, law enforcement personnel, teachers, therapists, faith communities, casual groups, and even people who work in prisons and jails. A touchstone of the training is the importance of trying not to assume anything about people when you meet them.

In this context, we're talking about not assuming someone's gender or pronouns, but we try to extend it even further to remind trainees that they don't know many things about the people they meet just by looking at them from the outside.

The first time TGRCNM did a training in a prison setting, it was pretty scary. This unfamiliar situation felt like it could be filled with folks who were hostile to trans people and to our training. The session had barely started when one of the prison employees who was attending the training raised her hand to announce to the entire room that she was the proud parent of a trans teenager whom she loved dearly. What a great lesson that was! So, try to remember that allies and friends can come from places that may seem unlikely at first.

Chapter 12 has some detailed information about making friends and creating new connections, so read that chapter for suggestions on reaching out for support. As someone at the outset of your transition process, looking for support in spaces with transgender people and people who are known to be caring and accepting of trans folks is a great idea.

This doesn't mean you should only make transgender and non-binary friends from this point forward; it simply means this is a moment in your life when knowing other folks like you, and being able to ask questions, vent, and laugh, can feel incredibly affirming.

(continued)

(continued)

What are some good ways to look for connections? Check these out:

- **Trans or LGBTQ organizations:** You can use the internet, and any personal referrals you get, to find local or state organizations that can offer help. Some will have support groups that may be great for you.

- **Support groups:** You may find a support group through a local or state organization, but remember that national organizations also offer online support groups. Some state or regional groups, like the Transgender Resource Center of New Mexico, have Zoom access for their groups and welcome folks from outside their service area.

- **Faith communities:** Although the question of participating in a faith community or tradition makes some LGBTQ people anxious, for others it's an important and sustaining part of their life. Chapter 12 lays out some resources for transgender and non-binary people who are Christian, Jewish, Muslim, and Buddhist. Even if you're questioning your faith, or interested in practices that are new to you, checking out these communities may be a great way to meet people who are like you.

- **Meetup.com:** This website has thousands of social groups organized around different interests. Many are LGBTQ gatherings or based on gender groupings.

TIP

There are many good ways to try to make friends, and Chapter 12 may spark your imagination. Don't forget that you don't have to limit yourself to trans/non-binary or LGBTQ people or organizations. You may be interested in a meetup group that enjoys hiking, or a support group about being sober or dealing with grief, if either of those issues is applicable to you. Just make sure that you think about your safety in terms of coming out or being visibly trans.

REMEMBER

You may be too anxious to try to meet people in real life at this point. That's okay! Your anxiety may decrease as you move through your gender transition, and if it doesn't, you can consult with a mental health provider about it. In the meantime, many transgender and non-binary people have found connections and relationships online. Check out Chapter 12 for more information.

Handling personal questions

As you push more deeply into your journey, you may encounter people who want to ask you questions about being transgender or non-binary. Each trans person has different boundaries in general, as well as specific boundaries for discussing their transgender or non-binary status and transition. No matter what your comfort level with inquiries is, you should never have to answer any question about your genitals, surgical history, sexual behavior, family planning, or reproductive choices. Those are deeply personal topics, and you don't have to respond to such requests for information, even if they're sincere.

With the huge range of other questions people may ask, it's really up to you to decide whether, when, and how to engage. It's a good idea to have a resource at your fingertips that you can refer curious people to. We're big believers in high-quality, in-person education about transgender and non-binary people. It's one of the three main aspects of our work at TGRCNM. But depending on where you live, you may not have a similar educational resource nearby. Plus, the person you're having the conversation with may have limited time or little attention for knowing more about trans folks. So, some simple online resources that link to more in-depth options are terrific.

One good resource is the web page "Questionable Questions about Transgender Identity" (https://tinyurl.com/4bsyby44) from Advocates for Trans Equality (A4TE), one of the foremost transgender advocacy organizations in the United States. Even if you're up for answering some questions, you can steer someone to this page or something similar for more information.

WARNING

Other important considerations are your assessment of your safety and whether you believe the person asking questions is really sincere and open to information and discussion. If you don't believe you're safe, your most crucial concern should be getting away from the situation without suffering any harm. The second issue is whether having a dialogue with the person serves any substantial purpose. If the curious person is someone you need to regularly interact with, you may assess the situation differently than if it's someone you aren't likely to ever see again.

Some people may be *eroticizing* or even *fetishizing* you — meaning they see you solely as a sexual object and want to interact in that way. That's probably not a situation where you want to be vulnerable or attempt to educate the person with your answers.

Other people may "ask questions" as a cover to simply argue with you about the validity of transgender people or your transgender status. They may be setting up a situation where they can try to persuade you about their religious or political opposition to trans and non-binary people. Even though people who have hard-line attitudes against trans folks do sometimes change over time, it's not likely to happen in this conversation, at this moment. And you should never feel it's your job to change someone's mind, either way. This is a situation where that old phrase "pick your battles" really applies.

Setting boundaries

Depending on how you were socialized in terms of gender, you have picked up different strategies for setting boundaries and asking for what you want and need. But regardless of your demographic characteristics, in childhood and now, you were probably discouraged from speaking up for yourself in a lot of meaningful ways. That means this is something many people have to figure out how to do in a healthy way in adulthood. And it's not easy! So, here are some tips:

>> **Figure out your wants and needs.** This sounds simple, but it may not be. Taking time to look inside and examine what really matters to you, as opposed to things you're willing to compromise on, will help you know when you need to set a boundary about something.

>> **Ask for help.** Getting the close people in your life to assist you in the boundary-setting process can be invaluable. These folks know you best and care about you. They can probably help you see when you may be ignoring yourself or going against what you need.

>> **Practice setting boundaries.** It's good to start small, with something you feel more comfortable asking for. This will be hard at first, so be prepared for some successes and some failures along the way

>> **Notice when your boundary has been crossed.** This may feel like anger or resentment, but you have to start connecting the dots on the emotional and physical sensations you have when something or someone crosses your boundaries.

>> **Don't overexplain.** It can be tempting to want to offer too many words and too much justification for setting a boundary. Most people respond better to simple, clear, kind communication. A great example of a straightforward response is something like, "Thank you so much for inviting me. I know you were probably looking forward to having the whole family together, but I've decided I won't be able to make it this time. I'd be happy to make a trip there next summer or get together next time you're in town."

REMEMBER

A boundary can't be something that you want someone else to do; it's a line that you draw for yourself. So even in the example above, it's unrealistic to expect the person not to invite you in the first place. Your boundary is that you decide not to go in order to take care of yourself.

TIP

You can find more great tips on how to offer simple explanations for maintaining your boundaries in "The 4 Steps to Saying No: How to set boundaries for your peace of mind" (https://tinyurl.com/5n7bdwdc).

Dealing With People Who Aren't Supportive

At this moment in history, dealing with a lack of support for gender transition is probably more the rule than the exception. For some lucky transgender and non-binary people, the only opposition comes from strangers, people "out there" who either don't believe that trans folks are real or believe that access and safety should be taken away from trans people. But for many, the challenges will be closer to home.

Transgender and non-binary people often report losing friends, partners, and family members when they come out or transition. This is a really painful and difficult situation for many people, and there's no correct way to deal with it. In fact, at the time of writing, lack of support is thought to be one of the primary reasons people turn back from transition (currently called *detransitioning*). Hopefully, in the near future, trans and non-binary people will be able to figure out who they are, take the steps they know are necessary to fully realize themselves, *and* stay closely connected to their loved ones. Today, though, this is still something people have to navigate on their gender journey.

First and foremost, see the earlier section "Setting boundaries." When people you love and want to stay in a relationship with aren't supportive, you have to figure out where your boundaries lie. Each trans person is going to have different boundaries, so try not to be too judgmental of your own choices and those of other trans and non-binary folks you know. Your boundaries are allowed to change over time, and with intention and practice, you'll get better at setting and holding them.

You may decide you don't want to cut important people out of your life, and there isn't much certain people can do that would cause you to completely sever the relationship. Parents and children often fall into this category. On the other hand, you may feel like people in your family or close friend group are truly disrespecting you after you come out to them, and you need to step away from them, temporarily or permanently. In this impossible situation, having supportive people to talk to about your transition process and your feelings can help you in your decision-making. But in the end, only you can determine what's healthiest for you in your relationships, today and as things shift and change in the future.

REMEMBER

It can't be said enough that life is (hopefully) long, and things can and will change. In our work, we've seen a lot of families reconcile after a period of separation, and we've seen long-term romantic relationships last through transitions or collapse. Sometimes these deeply painful changes make way for something different and also beautiful. And sometimes you may find other kinds of healing in the future.

Take care of yourself! Hold onto any connections that are supportive of you, and do what you can to forge new caring relationships (check out Chapters 12 and 13 for some good help with this).

WARNING

It's really ugly to talk about, but some trans and non-binary people face the threat of physical violence from people they know and thought cared about them. In the 2022 U.S. Transgender Survey, of the more than 92,000 respondents surveyed

>> More than one in ten (11 percent) of adult respondents who grew up in the same household with family, guardians, or foster parents said that a family member was violent toward them because they're transgender, and 8 percent were kicked out of the house because they're transgender.

>> Five percent of 16- and 17-year-olds who grew up in the same household with family, guardians, or foster parents said that a family member was violent toward them because they're transgender, and 1 percent were kicked out of the house because they're transgender.

TIP

At TGRCNM, we work with an organization in New Mexico called Resolve (https://resolvenm.org/), which is a chapter of IMPACT Violence Prevention (https://www.impactselfdefense.org/). This amazing program builds skills around a range of personal safety and violence prevention strategies and techniques. They start with boundary setting and awareness, provide information about violence and how it happens, and then show you how to ward off a physical attack. It isn't an easy class to take, but all TGRCNM staff take it together annually. The IMPACT chapters around the country often have scholarship programs, and we can't recommend it highly enough for transgender and non-binary kids and adults.

Another good strategy is working with friends or other community members to create safety plans. You can do things like

>> Implement a buddy system as much as possible. Make sure that people aren't out alone but travel in pairs or larger groups.

>> Share plans with each other and check in to make sure folks are okay and have arrived home after they're out with someone new.

>> Share your location with a small group through one of the location-sharing apps you can download to your phone so you can always track someone down if you haven't heard from them.

>> Share your legal name with at least one trusted person, so they can search for you in different locations, such as the hospital or jail, if you're too late returning from plans with someone.

Again, this is tough stuff to discuss, but having safety plans in place, and especially getting training from an organization like Resolve/IMPACT, can help if you're in a bad scenario with someone who wants to hurt you for being trans.

Making the Necessary Name and Legal Changes

Chapter 5 is your pocket guide to changing your name and updating your legal documents, so be sure to check out that chapter. Here, we provide an overview of the top-level legal shifts you may choose to make as part of your gender transition.

Taking on a new name

For a whole lot of transgender and non-binary people, a new name that's a better reflection of who they are is a huge step in the transition process. Although plenty of names in lots of different languages are neutral in terms of gender, many names convey some type of gender stereotype to the people around you. Chapter 5 has complete instructions about how to engage in the legal name change process, but how do you choose a new name in the first place?

Some transgender and non-binary people have been dreaming of a certain name since they were a kid. If you've always felt that a particular name was the perfect fit for you, that's great! You can probably just adopt that name and try it out for a little bit before you get into the legal process. If you're less positive about your new name, here are some ways you can narrow it down:

>> **Ask your family.** If you have a relationship with your family of origin, you can check with them to see whether they were considering any alternate names if you had been designated a different sex. Especially if you were born prior to the ultrasound era, your parents may have had a short list of "boy names" and "girl names." If you're non-binary, you can still be inspired by these names. And, of course, not all non-binary people want or need *androgynous* (gender-neutral) names.

>> **Check popular names from your birth year.** The Social Security Administration has a web page that lists the most popular baby names by decade (https://www.ssa.gov/oact/babynames/decades/). If you like any of the popular names during the decade you were born, it can help you make your decision.

>> **Look to nature, fiction, the gaming world, and so on.** People can find their new name from characters in their favorite books, movies, or video games. You may love or admire a fictional character whose name is a good fit. Your new name can come from anywhere.

>> **Keep your original name.** There are woman named Daryl (Hannah), Glenn (Close), and Joey (King). There are men named Channing (Tatum), Lindsey (Buckingham), and Rainn (Wilson). If you strongly desire a stereotypical masculine or feminine name, you aren't alone. A lot of trans people have waited their whole life to have a name that more specifically places them within a gender category. But if you love your first name, you shouldn't feel obligated to let it go. Plus, some folks are given androgynous names at birth, like Terry, Pat, Chris, and even Adrien!

>> **Name yourself for an important family member.** If someone in your family loved and supported you as a young person, renaming yourself for them is an incredible way to honor them and your relationship.

>> **Experiment with various names.** One of the best ways to check out new names is to try them out in everyday use. You can make a list of a few finalist names, and then let your friends, family, colleagues, or any other people you regularly interact with know that you're giving these names a trial run. Hearing them in different contexts, and from different people, may help you select the one you want to use going forward.

Changing your legal documents

Chapter 5 is a full road map of the legal documents you may need to change as part of your transition, especially if you change your legal name. In this section, you find a basic list that may look overwhelming. There's no question that transition isn't always easy, and some of the pieces take more time, energy, and commitment than others. Don't let this scare you off, though. Check out Chapter 5 for much more detail on how to change your legal documents, and utilize any resources you can find in your area, or barring that, nationally.

Some of the main legal documents you may need to update are

>> School records

>> Employee records

>> Bank, loan, and credit card documents

>> Health records

>> Insurance documents

- » State ID or driver's license
- » Birth certificate
- » Social Security records
- » Passport
- » Military records
- » Immigration records

Understanding Your Evolving Sexuality

For many transgender and non-binary people, transition is a time when their sexuality shifts and changes. For others, it may not change that much at all. Over time we've heard a lot of anecdotal accounts of folks who had sexual partners of only one gender prior to transition, and then had attractions and encounters with different kinds of partners once they began their transition. It may very well be that these people had different attractions all along but weren't able to have, or weren't able to be interested in, sex with certain partners before transition, when they were still being perceived as the wrong gender. A 2020 study on sexual orientation in transgender people (https://pubmed.ncbi.nlm.nih.gov/33483604/) came to the following conclusion:

> Sexual orientation did not change over time. We did not observe associations with serum levels of sex steroids or gender-affirming surgery (chest or genital surgery). Sexual orientation did not change during hormonal transition and was not associated with sex steroids or surgery. Also, preferences matched the partner's sexual identity. We do not assume that changing serum levels of sex steroids is directly associated with changes in partner choice. The number of people with a current partner increased, possibly due to the indirect effects of gender-affirming care.

We cover hormone therapy in detail in Chapter 8, but the use of gender-affirming hormones can definitely affect the *libido* (sex drive). Starting to take hormones at the typical masculinizing or feminizing doses brings on puberty, so the first few years of hormone therapy may involve unfamiliar experiences around sexuality. A lot of trans masculine people report levels of sexual desire and arousal that may be challenging to deal with. And the feminizing hormone regimen causes

- » Decreased sperm production
- » Decreased testicular volume
- » Less frequent spontaneous erections

These all typically contribute to lower libido for trans feminine people. But each person is different, and if this feels like a problem rather than a relief, talk to your healthcare provider about options for boosting your libido.

You may still be figuring out your orientation, and that's absolutely fine. This isn't something you have to lock down today, or ever. Questioning your gender or sexuality is a normal part of life. Plus, actualizing yourself in your real gender may not change whom you're attracted to (or it may feel like it opens doors for you in that area), but either way, you may find yourself more open to your body and your sexuality, and to exploring your own pleasure and desire.

If you're trying to figure all this out, know that these days, many different orientations have been identified (https://www.healthline.com/health/different-types-of-sexuality). A sampling of orientation words includes the following:

>> **Asexual:** Not experiencing sexual desire for others (this doesn't mean that these folks don't like people, or even that they never have sex)

>> **Bisexual:** Attracted to two or more genders

>> **Gay:** Attracted to the same gender (sometimes used to specifically talk about men who are attracted to men)

>> **Lesbian:** Women attracted to women

>> **Pansexual:** Attracted to individual people without regard to their gender or genitals

>> **Polysexual:** Attracted to various, but not necessarily all, genders

>> **Queer:** A descriptor that many LGBTQ people use as an empowering word, also with a political aspect

>> **Straight:** Attracted to the opposite gender

Recognizing the Long-Term Commitments of Transition

When anyone undertakes changes this big, they won't be the only one touched by all the ripples that spread out from them. All the people and relationships around you are going to be affected. This will probably be a mixed bag, not just a tough one. Keep in mind that you'll encounter some bright spots along the way, too!

Taking charge of relationships

It isn't always easy to steer your ship through the rough waters of a gender transition, and managing your relationships is one important aspect of this journey. Many people have a strong desire to preserve their connections with their kids, partners, parents, and siblings. Although you won't have complete control over the outcomes, it's worth considering how you want to handle these folks in your life.

Your children

Being honest and communicating in developmentally appropriate ways are both crucial components to getting through this together. Reassuring them that you are the same person and will always be their parent can help, and you absolutely want to listen patiently and openly to any feelings they have. If they're scared or resistant, it can feel like rejection, so be sure to prepare yourself to hear those things for what they are: part of your child's process. These ideas and more are covered in a great guide from the FOLX Health website which also features a reading list (https://tinyurl.com/4fvycpus).

TIP

If you're comfortable, it can help kids to be allowed to keep calling you by whatever term of endearment they've used previously, even if it's something like Mama or Dad. If you feel that makes you unsafe out in public, or it's just too hard on your *gender dysphoria* (discomfort or distress caused by your sex and gender not being aligned), that's completely understandable. But some trans and non-binary folks feel fine hearing these familiar words from their children, and the kids can feel validated by it.

Your partner (or partners)

Coming out to a partner is often a distinctly scary prospect. The fear of losing your beloved can make you want to hold back from being open about what's going on with you. While that can be tempting, it often ends up causing even more unintentional hurt. And you don't have any way to know how things are going to resolve for you and your current partner, or partners.

It's true that relationships sometimes don't have the same form on both sides of a transition. That doesn't mean you can't have a loving connection with anyone you're involved with now, even if it's different from the way you're connected today. People fear shifts and changes in their relationships, but something even better may be out there for you if you can embrace your gender journey and give complete, honest info to anyone you're dating.

You may be afraid that you'll never find romantic love as a trans or non-binary person. Dating definitely does have its pitfalls for trans folks, but some great person (or people) will be able to see you for who you are. Staying in an unhealthy relationship will keep any future happiness out of your reach.

Your parents and siblings

You may really want the approval and acceptance of the people who raised you and the people you grew up with. On the other hand, you may have a complicated relationship with these folks, or you may have already cut ties with them. If you're hoping to stay in contact with your parents and siblings, you may be agonizing about how to disclose what you're figuring out about your gender and your path forward. Here are some tips:

>> **Take a temperature check.** You can casually try to find out more about how your family feels about transgender and non-binary people by asking questions or bringing up current events or trans celebrities. Gauging their reactions may give you an idea about their attitudes on the subject.

>> **Prepare for the conversation.** You can prepare for coming out to your family in a few ways. You'll probably want to organize your thoughts and what you want to say. Having some key talking points and sticking to your own experience can keep you from getting too rocked if your folks pepper you with questions or have defensive reactions.

Ask your support people to check in with you at an appointed time if you're going to come out in person. Earlier in the chapter, we provide some chilling stats about trans folks who experienced violence from family members (see "Dealing with people who aren't supportive" earlier in this chapter). If you aren't totally sure how your family will react, check out that section for some tips on preparing for a violent reaction.

>> **Practice the conversation.** Practicing any important communication can boost your confidence and help you stay steady in the heat of the actual moment of the conversation. You can practice in the mirror, record yourself with your phone and watch it, or ask your support folks to role-play with you.

>> **Set boundaries.** Read the section earlier in this chapter about boundary setting (see "Setting boundaries") and be ready to hold your boundaries throughout the process of coming out. Family members may have a lot of really big feelings about your announcement and your transition process, and it can be hard to let them work through their feelings without taking it personally. You're allowed to take a break or skip some family events to take care of yourself, while still staying in a relationship with your family members.

>> **Make sure you have support.** Gather up all your resources! Join a support group and talk to your friends about coming out. A therapist can be a huge

help. It's also a great idea to try to figure out who will be the most supportive person in your family and start with them.

>> **Choose your method.** Don't be embarrassed if you decide to send a letter rather than having any conversations in person. This goes back to your boundaries, and it can also allow you to be more articulate in expressing your experiences and feelings. How you come out to your family is up to you.

>> **Have patience and extend grace.** If you come out to your family and they react violently, your safety is the only important concern. But if the situation goes pretty well, or even if their reactions are mixed but you want to give them some time to see how things evolve, it's a big deal when you can extend grace and patience to your loved ones as they figure out their thoughts and feelings, which *always* involves making mistakes. This doesn't mean that you must cross or ignore your own boundaries, but trying not to be too harsh with your corrections and reminders can go a long way.

Your extended family

Relationships with extended family are diverse and complicated. Just like with immediate family members, some people have close, vibrant relationships with cousins, aunts, uncles, grandparents, great-grandparents, and other distant relatives. But some trans people barely know these folks, and won't feel any obligation to share this part of their life.

If your relationships with extended family members hold a lot of meaning for you, then you can use the section immediately preceding this one for some tips on how to come out to them about what's happening to you. Or you can rely on your immediate family members as buffers to either start this conversation with your extended family or even be your primary messengers.

FIVE TIPS FOR COMING OUT AS TRANSGENDER IN IMMIGRANT FAMILIES

Navigating a conversation about your transgender identity with family members from immigrant backgrounds can be complex. Cultural differences, language barriers, and generational perspectives often add layers to the process. Here are some strategies shared by members of the LGBTQ community:

- **Build a support system.** Reach out to friends, chosen family, or online support groups to ground yourself emotionally before, during, and after your conversation.

(continued)

(continued)

- **Speak their language.** If possible, use your parents' native language to explain your identity. Seeking out translated resources can help bridge any gaps in understanding.

- **Introduce representation.** Connecting family members with other transgender people — through personal meetings, media, or support organizations — can normalize transgender experiences for them.

- **Manage your expectations.** Acceptance doesn't always mean full understanding. Meet your loved ones where they are, acknowledging their learning process.

- **Be patient.** Change takes time. Approach conversations slowly and steadily, allowing space for questions and growth.

For more insights on coming out, explore the resources at https://folxhealth.com.

Seeing how transition affects work and school

Work and school are places where many people spend big portions of their life. You may be transitioning on the job or while you're at school. Some people have no choice but to go through their transition process in the midst of people they knew before and will still be constantly associating with during and after they get into whatever steps they're taking. Others time things so that they're ending some chapters and starting new ones when they're transitioning.

For example, some folks have moved to a new city during transition so they're more anonymous. But no matter how you figure out this piece of your transition, you'll need to account for group settings like work or school.

Your workplace

The Human Rights Campaign's website has a guide to coming out at work, a guide to trans-inclusive benefits, and a review of workplace discrimination laws and policies (https://www.hrc.org/resources/workplace?topic=transgender). If your workplace has a formal human resources representative or department, you should go to them as soon as you can to report that you're beginning the transition process. Letting them know means they can assist you, and it also provides documentation that your workplace knows you're transgender or non-binary, as well as the timeline for your transition. If you're protected by state nondiscrimination laws, this documentation can be valuable should you feel you're experiencing discrimination during the process.

Depending on the size of your workplace, how many coworkers you have, and the demographic diversity of your colleagues, you may have a difficult time with a majority of them, or you may be coming out into a supportive and accepting environment. People may object to you using the bathroom that matches your gender, or they may pick up your new name and pronouns with almost no bumps at all.

Check out the section "Setting Boundaries" earlier in this chapter, because this will be important during this time. Having good boundaries that protect you doesn't mean being hostile or aggressive. It simply means refusing to allow coworkers to disrespect you or do you harm at work.

Even if you think your supervisor won't be supportive, you'll probably need to go to them first if you experience mistreatment from colleagues. Following the chain of reporting at your job is another good step for establishing documentation for any future legal action, and it can prevent blame from landing on you for not following the correct procedure.

REMEMBER

You don't have to be a professional trans educator. If your coworkers have a lot of questions, you can point them to good online resources or, even better, local high-quality trans education. One good option comes from our friends at A4TE (https://transequality.org/trans-101), and another is GLAAD's Here We Are campaign (https://www.herewearenow.com/).

At TGRCNM, we are big believers in informing people about trans and non-binary people and the issues they face. We've been called in many times to provide workplace training when someone has just come out as trans or non-binary.

Over and over, we've received reports that the workforce in these places gained knowledge and awareness about trans people and shifted their attitudes and behaviors toward their trans coworker, or trans people in general. Being able to bring a great trans trainer into your workplace may help move things in a positive direction.

Over time, some of the initial pressure points can smooth out, even on their own. The uneasiness some of your coworkers may express can ebb as they get to know the real you. The newness will wear off, and people will see that you still just go into the restroom to use the bathroom and wash your hands. As they experience this for themselves, don't be surprised if it becomes less of an issue.

WARNING

If you aren't able to make any headway and you truly feel you're experiencing discrimination or abuse, you may have a lawsuit on your hands. Unfortunately, these suits are difficult to win because of how hard it can be to prove discrimination or mistreatment based on a protected category. Plus, your state has to have laws that protect trans people in the first place.

So, most importantly, get out of the situation if you can. Try to find a new job and leave any place where you're treated disrespectfully or unlawfully. Economically, this may be difficult or impossible for you. Get whatever help you can to find out if you have any legal options and whether any resources may exist to help you file a complaint and/or find a new job.

Some trans/non-binary folks choose not to come out at all in a job if they truly believe they could be harmed or fired. This is often due to needing the income from that job. Definitely start trying to find something new, where you can be yourself. But if you feel like you will not be safe coming out, and you also cannot simply leave the job you are in, trust your instincts.

Your school environment

School environments are very much like workplace environments in how unpredictable they can be for trans and non-binary people who are coming out or are unable to blend in during and after their transition.

Some schools have protective policy in place and even have Gender Sexuality Alliance or Gay Straight Alliance clubs and *Safe Space* programs (offices or classrooms where students can talk to an adult in a nonjudgmental environment, receive support, and get connected to resources). Figure 3-1, from the Albuquerque Public Schools website, is an example of what Safe Zone or Safe Space signs may look like.

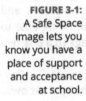

FIGURE 3-1:
A Safe Space image lets you know you have a place of support and acceptance at school.

If your school feels unsupportive, or even hostile, your safest bet may be to try to find as much support as you can in and out of school, and ride out your time there as best you can. Make an effort to search out one supportive teacher, faculty member, or staff person.

Keep an eye out for other students who have interests like yours or seem approachable. TGRCNM has a youth group, so we've heard a lot of stories about friends sustaining someone through the years they had to spend in an unfriendly school.

You may also feel the pull toward advocacy. If you want to try to change your school environment, Lambda Legal has a guide called "Bending the Mold" (https://tinyurl.com/7fh24exv), which has great resources for everyone, even if you aren't going to lead the proverbial charge. A4TE lists a bunch of other resources that may be helpful, including model school policy and know-your-rights materials (https://transequality.org/issues/education).

Living a low- or no-disclosure life

Some trans and non-binary people are able to visually blend in and limit how out they choose to be. They may restrict their disclosure about being trans to very close people and keep their truth from others, at work or school or elsewhere in their life.

In our trainings we talk about being *visibly trans*, or whether or not you're able to assimilate, or fit in, visually. Historically, this has been referred to as *passing*, and folks who choose to blend in all the time are *stealth*.

These terms — especially passing — have some issues.

First, the word *passing* has a lot of racial history, because it has been used to describe folks of color blending in as white, with a lot of accompanying danger if they're discovered.

Lumping that history in with the history of trans people (of all racial backgrounds) blending in takes you down the slippery slope of comparing the hardships of two traits that have both been oppressed — and which overlap.

Also, trans and non-binary people aren't pretending to be the gender they are. They aren't deceiving people into believing they're something they're not. They are finally actualizing themselves as the people they truly are, and showing it to the outside world.

Whether you choose to assimilate or not is totally up to you (and your transition process, genetic luck, and other factors). A whole lot of trans and non-binary people before you have lived (or hidden) their truth in every possible way.

2
Managing Social Transition

IN THIS CHAPTER

» Shifting your look with new clothes

» Adopting new hairstyles and looks

» Packing and tucking

» Utilizing a binder

» Using common prostheses

Chapter **4**

Changing Your Style and Appearance

We know that not all transgender and non-binary people experience gender dysphoria (a disconnect between the sex assigned at birth and their internal sense of gender) or want to take hormones or undergo surgery. That doesn't mean they don't necessarily want to shift their appearance, for their personal gratification and/or to be perceived accurately by people around them. In this chapter, you discover ways you can modify your appearance that aren't medical steps. These strategies can supplement medical transition care, or you can do them on their own.

Whether you intend to pursue medical transition or not, you can use this chapter to explore the landscape of clothing, hair, and makeup. You can also look into packing, tucking, and binding (all ways to minimize the appearance of certain body parts), and the use of prosthetic devices that are common to the transgender experience.

Managing Clothing and Grooming Changes

For many people, changing the way they dress and present themselves can be a big adjustment. For some folks, getting a new haircut that more accurately reflects their internal gender to the world can be the first step in a long personal journey that involves many steps, including medical treatments (see Part 3), social adaptations (see Chapter 12), and legal processes (see Chapter 5). For others, changing their hair, asking people to call them by a new name, or adopting a new style of dress can be *the* step they need to take to feel more fulfilled in their gender. Your path is your own, and nobody is more transgender or non-binary, or more of a man or a woman, because of the transition journey they take.

Adapting your clothing

Although buying a new wardrobe may sound like fun, it can also be expensive and intimidating. Borrowing clothes, shopping at thrift stores, and participating in clothing exchanges are always great ways to switch up your style at a low cost, but these strategies can be especially useful as you figure out what you like and how you want to be seen by others.

TIP

When you were a child, you may not have been free to express your gender in the way that's authentic to you. If that was the case, you probably had limited opportunities to explore or embrace styles that you love. Don't be embarrassed to create a *vision board*, or file of looks you admire or want to try out. You can find tons of websites with street style photos and even pop culture media that may inspire looks you love.

Some transgender and non-binary people have always dressed in a way that reflected their true internal gender. In those cases, the adjustments they make to their appearance may be minor, or even unnecessary. In any case, here are some points to keep in mind as you explore potential changes to how you dress:

>> **Consider the fit.** If you're going to have hormone treatments or surgery, the way your clothes fit can change dramatically. You may find that you wear a different size than you're used to, or the way you tailor your clothing may change. We've even heard of folks whose shoe size changed when they began medical transition.

>> **Notice whether your clothes are fine as is.** If you've already been dressing in a way that feels like a reflection of your true self and you're not interested in medical transition, then congratulations. You probably don't want or need to adjust your clothes right now. Of course, your style may change over time, and you may enjoy trying out different looks from time to time for many different reasons.

>> **Embrace the appearance of the gender you feel.** If you've been trying to hide your gender, experimenting with clothes that feel more in line with who you are will be a tender, and maybe scary, experience. For information about accessing support for your journey, see Part 4.

You should feel absolutely free to experiment with whatever clothes and styles appeal to you, especially if you've always wanted to wear certain things but were restricted from trying them out.

Know that you're not alone if you've believed that you had to hide who you are. And enjoy the sense of freedom and relief that comes from finally letting yourself move forward to presenting in a more authentic way!

For some folks, fitting into different masculine and feminine stereotypes is a high priority. If this is true for you, then you may want to consider the following factors as you plan any clothing adjustments:

>> **Your age:** Conventions about how to dress change as people get older. If fitting in is something you value, then observing and researching what's considered age-appropriate can help you blend in.

>> **Your profession:** The job you do can dictate, to some extent, the clothes that are appropriate and/or functional for you to wear. Even though wearing high heels is a fun new adventure for some trans folks, stilettos may not be the best footwear choice for working at a home improvement store or driving a truck!

>> **Your activity:** By the same token, you can be a little more adventurous if you're going out to a club with friends or taking a vacation. *Cisgender* folks (whose gender matches their designated sex at birth) use these opportunities to try out new looks, too!

>> **Your surroundings:** What's considered stereotypically masculine or feminine clothing is different if you live in a rural farming community rather than a highly populated urban area. Other demographic factors also affect how different gender expressions are viewed. You've probably spent some time observing the people in your community, so you know a lot about how they measure and display gender in their clothing choices. You can use that knowledge as a guidepost as you move forward. Trust yourself.

TIP

For some folks, even trying out these new clothes in private can be a huge deal. Trying on gender-specific clothing in the privacy of your room or home can feel like real freedom. Another private option (if you're not ready for everyone to see you still) is putting some items on under the clothes your currently wearing.

TIP

Jewelry is another fun way to express yourself. You don't have to stick to stereotypically masculine or feminine choices. Playing around and trying new pieces and different styles is a great way to find out what you like on yourself.

Choosing a hairstyle

Feeling like a man, a woman, or a non-binary person may inspire you to change your hair. But remember that cisgender people wear their hair in every conceivable style and length: Cisgender men may have long hair, and cisgender women may have short hair. That means you don't have to conform to a specific hairstyle in order to be valid in your gender.

TIP

For some trans and non-binary people, it's important to have a haircut that telegraphs their membership in the lesbian, gay, bisexual, and transgender (LGBT) communities. Asking someone who wears their hairstyle proudly can lead you to a stylist you love who caters to LGBT people. Also, observing people around you and checking out websites and online photo galleries can give you ideas about new styles to try out.

For people who want a more stereotypically masculine or feminine look, a change in hairstyle can mean going to a barber or a beauty parlor or salon for the first time. Even though this is exciting, it's another new experience that comes with challenges.

If possible, try to identify a barber or stylist who is friendly and knowledgeable about transgender and non-binary people. For ideas about how to find supportive salons or barbershops, see Chapter 12.

Hair extensions and wigs are also great options for a lot of folks. Especially if you are trans feminine and have experienced any pattern balding, extensions or wigs may give you confidence when you're interacting with others.

Experimenting with cosmetics or shaving practices

For trans women, trans feminine people, and some non-binary folks, experimenting with makeup is a creative step toward expressing their gender. We've even known some transgender men and trans masculine people who enjoy makeup or perform as drag queens. Never forget that your gender journey and your relationship to your gender are your own, and your choices can't be wrong!

If cosmetics appeal to you, it can be deeply affirming to purchase makeup and get some initial tips and ideas from a retail outlet that's friendly to trans and non-binary people. Jecca Blac (https://us.jeccablac.com/) specializes in makeup for trans folks, and Sephora (www.sephora.com) has a history of hosting trans makeup classes and engaging in other outreach to trans and non-binary people.

TIP

If you live in a rural area without easy access to help with your makeup choices, you can find lots of makeup tutorials on YouTube. And both Jecca Blac and Sephora sell their products online.

Shaving can also be a gender-affirming grooming practice for many trans and non-binary people. Shaving is a nonpermanent way to remove hair from all over the body and face, and it's a long-term hair removal solution for some people. Some people may begin shaving parts of their bodies that they haven't shaved before.

Other temporary hair removal strategies are waxing and *depilatory creams* (products that are applied like lotion and remove hair from the face or body). You may eventually seek more permanent hair removal solutions, such as electrolysis and laser hair removal. Either way, proper shaving technique can cut down on irritation and reactions.

The American Academy of Dermatology provides these tips for a clean shave, which you can also find online (www.aad.org/public/everyday-care/skin-care-basics/hair/how-to-shave):

>> **Wet your skin before you begin.** Shaving dry can be painful and damage your skin. A great time to shave is right after a shower, because your skin will be clean, moist, and exfoliated, which can help prevent blades from clogging up.

>> **Apply shaving cream or gel.** A product for sensitive skin can be helpful for people who deal with that issue. A soothing aftershave balm or lotion is a great tool for moisturizing and nourishing the skin, too.

>> **Shave in the direction your hair grows.** Doing this can cut down on skin bumps and razor burn.

>> **Rinse after each swipe of the razor.** Rinsing the blades helps keep them sharp and gets rid of debris that can attract bacteria.

>> **Replace your razor or your blades regularly.** While recommendations vary, most experts suggest changing out your blades sometime between 5 and 10 shaves. You can watch for signs that the blades need to be changed sooner, such as a feeling of dullness, difficult-to-remove residue between blades, or visible rust.

>> **Store your razor in a dry area.** Allowing the razor to dry completely can prevent bacterial growth.

REMEMBER

Taking testosterone, or T, will grow new hair on your face, but shaving can still feel like a really affirming thing to do. Whether or not you intend to start T at some point, if shaving gives you gender euphoria, do it!

You can use cosmetics to essentially draw a beard or hair on your face. Spirit gum and hair clippings are another way to get a realistic-looking beard. Both methods are old drag king tricks, so you can find many amazing tutorials online. You can have fun experimenting, or use one of these tricks consistently to obtain the look you want.

Modifying Your Body Profile: Considering the Possibilities

One of the benefits of cross-sex hormone therapy is that it changes the contours of most people's bodies. Testosterone concentrates fat deposits in the belly and away from the hips and thighs, for example. Estrogen causes breast growth for most folks. (To get the details about hormone therapy, go to Chapter 8.) But don't despair if you aren't interested in medical transition. As any experienced drag queen will tell you, there are other ways to change the look of your body's silhouette.

Trying out packing

Prosthetic penises are often associated with transgender men, but some non-binary folks also feel more comfortable and confident when they use a *packer* (a silicone prosthetic and/or padding over or around the genitalia to create the appearance that a penis is present under clothing). Regardless of your gender, feel free to experiment with *packing* (the process of placing the packer).

Packers come in a few different styles, so research different online vendors and types of packers to see what appeals to you. You can find these types of packers:

>> **Aesthetic only:** These packers are made to create a more realistic bulge around the crotch and are used just for appearance.

>> **Functional for urinating:** Other packers are made to enable to you to stand up when you pee. They're usually called stand-to-pee devices (or STPs).

>> **Sexually effective:** Some packers are designed to be effective for use during penetrative sex.

These days quite a few websites offer high-quality packers in all these styles. You can try out more than one; just be aware that they aren't cheap.

You may find that your regular underwear works great with your packer, but if not, many vendors also sell special underwear designed to hold a packer. These are usually typical men's underwear with a special pocket sewn into the inside that prevents the packer from moving around. Some folks have pretty embarrassing stories about their packer escaping their underwear and working its way down their pants leg. Don't let that scare you, though. Just practice with your new packer at home — and with different kinds of underwear — until you feel sure of it and yourself.

Adjusting with tucking

For folks who were born with a penis, tucking can be a great option for creating a smoother crotch appearance, removing a visible bulge from your profile. You have different options for tucking: using tape, wearing a *gaff* or *tucking underwear* (compression underwear that flattens the lower body and pelvic area), or just putting on tight underwear and layering your clothes.

If you're wondering what *tucking* means, it's basically the process of securing the penis and/or testicles between the legs to create a smooth front. It can also involve gently pushing the testicles into the spaces in the pelvis known as the *inguinal canals*. You don't need to have gender dysphoria to appreciate the appearance achieved by tucking.

The steps for tucking are

1. **Gather your supplies.**

    You'll need tape (tucking tape is made for this purpose and is available for purchase online — but kinesiology tape is a close match), a gaff, tight underwear, or a combination.

    You can cut the tape into strips of the correct length before you begin the process. You'll learn the size of the strips you need by practicing. This will be different for different body types and sizes.

    You can shave or trim your pubic hair if you're using tape (see the previous section for shaving tips). This can prevent the tape from pulling your skin and hair when you remove it.

2. **If you're using a gaff or tight underwear, put them on and pull them halfway up your legs.**

3. **Use two or three fingers to push each testicle into the corresponding inguinal canal.**

    Take your time when you're first getting started. This should never be painful, so if you do feel pain, just take a breather and give it another try when the pain stops.

Some people don't push the testicles into the inguinal canals and instead just position them back and to the sides of their pelvic bones.

4. **Pull the penis and scrotum back between the legs.**

   If you're tucking the testicles, this will help hold them in place.

5. **Use two or three pieces of tape to hold the penis and scrotum in place.**

   Stretch the tape from the lower part of your stomach, about where the top of your underwear sits, over the shaft of the penis and over your butt to your tailbone.

   You can also use two pieces that extend from the shaft of the penis, beneath each butt cheek, and out to your hip. These would be going from the left side of your front to the left side of your back, not crossing over. Figure 4-1 illustrates the pattern the tape can take.

6. **Pull your underwear up.**

   A gaff, or special tucking underwear, can help you achieve a flatter appearance because it's made with a stiff panel in front. But using tight or compression underwear can also work well.

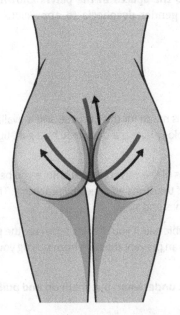

FIGURE 4-1:
This is the way the first pieces of tape can be positioned when you're tucking.

REMEMBER

Tucking is safe! You can take the following simple steps to ensure that you don't do any harm to your body when tucking:

- If you feel any pain, take a break.
- Be aware that a little discomfort is normal, especially when tucking is new to you.
- Try to use the bathroom before you tuck if you need to go.
- Don't use duct tape, scotch tape, or packing tape.
- Give your body a break from tucking. Sleeping is a great time to not tuck.
- Keep an eye out for the common side effects of tucking: itching, rash, testicular pain, skin infections, urinary tract infections, and pain in the penis.

WARNING

It's tempting to "hold it in" when you're tucking, but it's important to try to go to the bathroom when your body needs to. You'll need to remove your gaff, underwear, or tape and untuck in order to go. Once you're done, you can re-tuck. You can usually use tape two or three times before you need to replace it.

REMEMBER

Each person is different, so experiment with different methods to find what helps you feel most comfortable and confident. Trans women definitely report being able to get great results without tape or special undergarments.

Considering binding or chest compression options

Wearing a binder, or using other methods of compressing your chest, can be a great way to feel good about how you look, whether or not it's in conjunction with your gender.

Many trans masculine and non-binary people experience gender euphoria from these practices, though. You should be aware of a few things about binding and compression to get the best result and keep your body safe while you do it.

A *binder* is a tightly fitting undergarment that presses your chest down to create a more stereotypically masculine appearance. It looks like a tank top or undershirt, and it can be long enough to tuck into your pants, or it may end in the middle of your torso.

You pull some binders over your head, or you can step into them. Others are made with hook and eye or Velcro closures. You can find many excellent binders online.

TIP

Some people simply wear an old-fashioned sports bra or even layer a couple of tight-fitting shirts. If these tricks don't feel like they will work for you full time, they can be great strategies when you're giving your body a break from binding.

Finally, different types of tape work well for some people. Of course, we don't mean duct tape, packing tape, or masking tape! Kinesiology tape or elastic therapeutic tape are the way to go. You can also find a product called TransTape online (`https://transtape.life` — the site contains explicit images).

You don't have to have gender dysphoria to enjoy the look and feel of a flatter chest. If you want to give binding a try, go for it! Just keep it safe.

Binding and chest compression may cause injury if you don't do it safely. So, keep these safe binding tips in mind:

>> **If you can't take a deep breath, remove your binder.** Something is wrong if you're having trouble breathing. Shortness of breath may be a sign that you need a larger binder.

>> **Make sure you have full range of motion in your arms when binding.** You should be able to raise your arms over your head, and cross your arms in front of you like scissors when wearing your binder.

>> **Use only materials that are made for binding.** ACE bandages, plastic wrap, and tape not made for binding (like duct tape or masking tape) can harm your skin.

>> **Give your body a break.** You should try to take off your binder every 8–12 hours, and it's a great idea not to sleep in it (even though you may be tempted).

>> **Don't wear a binder that's too small.** This can be tempting, but it may not make your chest look flatter and can cause serious injury. The size guides provided by binder companies are the best way to try to get the right fit the first time you order. Don't be scared to return your binder for the correct size if you ordered the wrong one.

>> **Hand-wash and air-dry your binder regularly.** If you get more than one binder, you can wash and rotate them. Washing helps you prevent acne and keeps the binder from smelling ripe.

>> **Keep an eye out for the common side effects of binding.** These include back pain, soreness, chest pain, difficulty breathing, numbness, tingling, overheating, dehydration, and skin rash or irritation. Pay attention to your body, and talk to your medical provider, if you have one, if you experience any of these things.

If you have a bigger chest, it can be hard to get a fully flat look without surgery. Binding is great, and can help you feel more confident, for sure. But check out images of folks with your body type to see what your results might look like. Many of the online binder vendors have differently sized models on their websites.

REMEMBER

You have every right to present yourself in whatever way makes you feel good. It is important to remember, though, that everyone may not share your joy with your new look. This can include folks you already know and strangers out in the world. This is especially true if you are not able to blend in for any reason.

If people still perceive you as a woman, for example, they may have strong, but unconscious, expectations about you upholding the gender norms and stereotypes sometimes forced on women.

That doesn't obligate you to do it. It's just another consideration for you to take into account as you factor your needs, desires, and safety throughout this process.

Adding prostheses

People employ different prosthetic devices to change the shape of their bodies. Packers are prostheses that many folks love using (see "Trying out packing" earlier in this chapter).

In this section, we explore breast forms and hip/butt padding. Drag queens have known about these little gems for a long time. If you haven't heard of them, you may love looking into what's available.

Many online vendors sell breast prostheses and hip pads. Not all of them are specifically for transgender people, but they're still good places to purchase these items. Hip pads are usually made of foam and are attached with silicone adhesive, and some are built into shapewear undergarments. Figure 4-2 shows a typical version of the shapewear model.

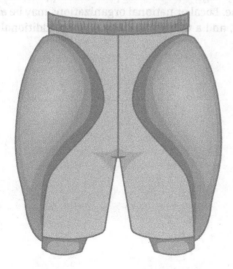

FIGURE 4-2: A photo of hip-padding shapewear.

Breast prostheses, or breast forms, come in a wide array of colors, shapes, and sizes. You wear them under a bra, and they should stay in place throughout the day. Online vendors have sizing guides and instructions to help you figure out which size to order.

Breast forms are made of silicone, and the different shapes mimic the appearance of different types of breasts. People who have wider chests may prefer triangular prostheses, while the oval ones can work better for folks with smaller chests. Figure 4-3 illustrates the two shapes.

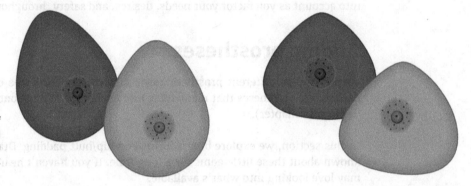

FIGURE 4-3:
A photo of oval (left) and triangular (right) silicone breast prostheses.

TIP

Point of Pride (https://www.pointofpride.org) is a well-known organization that provides free binders and free femme shapewear, as well as financial assistance for electrolysis, hormone therapy, and even surgery. They also offer financial aid for prostheses, fertility assistance, vocal training, and more.

But they aren't the only organization that provides support; new programs are being started all the time. Local or national organizations may be able to help with your transition journey, and a web search may turn up additional funding assistance programs.

Chapter **5**

Changing Legal Documents

Of the many changes you can make as you transition, choosing your name — should you decide to — can be among the most exciting. Your name is a defining aspect of your identity, and changing it is a big step. However, you should understand the important legal implications of having a new name and ensuring all your documentation aligns with your identity.

In this chapter we dive into what it takes to update your legal name and all your official documents, such as your birth certificate, state ID, and Social Security records. We also touch on the requirements for modifying your military and immigration records.

REMEMBER

Many transgender and non-binary people feel it's critical to align their legal documents with their true identity. Keep in mind that changing your legal records can have far-reaching consequences, including risks to your safety, employment, education, and other concerns. It's important to remember that the decision to make these changes is personal, like all the aspects of gender transition we cover in this book. And, just like other important elements of transition, changes to your legal records can be undertaken in combination with other steps or on their own.

So, don't be intimidated. Even though some of these tasks seem overwhelming, help is available if you need it. You can do it!

Updating Your Name

Changing your legal name is an exciting step for a lot of people. It can help you feel more authentic and in touch with your reality. But a name change ripples out into many areas of your life and forces you to update a lot of important records and other personal information. For example, some schools and employers require students and employees to use their legal name for their internal email address, and of course, paychecks and other work-related documents have to be executed in the employee's legal name.

If changing your name is part of your journey, you've come to the right place. For help picking out a new name, see Chapter 3. In the following sections, we cover the basic steps for making a legal name change and highlight the other documents you typically need to consider after the process is complete. It's vital to remember that these processes vary widely across the United States. We want to give you some helpful specifics, but nothing will replace thoroughly researching the processes that apply to you, in the relevant locations.

Knowing how to change your legal name

The law governing name changes, including the age at which they're considered an adult name change, is set at the state level, so you'll need to check the legal requirements in the state where you currently live. These varied legal requirements will cover things like which forms you have to fill out, how you will file, whether you have to publish your name change in the paper, and more. You always change your name in the judicial district or county you live in, not, for example, where you were born. The courts have their own websites, which often but not always provide copies of the documents you need and list the steps and requirements you must follow.

TIP

For many years, the best overall resource created by and for transgender people has been the ID Documents Center on the Advocates for Trans Equality (A4TE) website (https://transequality.org/documents). This terrific web page offers state-by-state resources for all the documents that we discuss in this chapter.

Again, the process varies depending on your location in the U.S., but here are some typical steps you must take to change your name:

1. **Fill out the name change forms.**

   You can most likely go to the district courthouse to obtain blank forms, but if that doesn't work for any reason, you can almost always find and download the forms online. Once you have a blank set of forms, make a copy and put them aside in case you make any errors filling them out the first time.

The primary form is the petition to change your name. You can fill in the blanks on most of these forms, but don't sign them. They probably need to be signed in front of a *notary public* (someone granted a special seal by the government to be able to sign documents as an impartial witness). This may seem like a lot of paperwork, but usually the questions are limited to your old name, new name, county of residence, Social Security number, and possibly the reason for your name change.

2. **File the forms.**

   You may need to have a notary sign your forms, and then you need to make a few copies, at least one extra set to keep; and again, different states have different requirements (even for little things like the number of copies!). Once the forms are filled out, you must file them with the court. Some courts accept electronic filing, so be sure to check whether you're required to file in person, especially if you live far away from your district or county courthouse.

3. **Wait for the review and official change.**

   At this point it falls to the judge to review your petition and grant your name change. Some states have streamlined this so it's nearly an administrative process. In those states, such as Oregon, you have to physically appear at a hearing only if the court sends you a hearing notice. However, many states still require a hearing in front of a judge to finalize a name change, in which case you'll receive a date for your hearing when you file your forms.

   You don't usually need to dress formally for a name change hearing, but it's a good idea to convey respect for the court and the judge by what you wear and how you present yourself.

   Barring any unforeseen issues, the judge should grant your name change, and you should receive a final order of name change. It's a great idea to grab a few certified copies if your hearing was at the courthouse. These can come in handy as you provide notice everywhere you need to.

4. **Provide notice.**

   Once your name change is complete, it's time to share the good news! This definitely means informing family, friends, colleagues, and anyone else you want to tell. You'll also want to provide official notice to several entities. We go more deeply into a few of them in the following sections, but it's important to consider

   - School

   - Employer

   - U.S. Postal Service (change of address form)

   - Banks and credit card companies

- Other lenders
- Insurance companies
- Utility and phone companies
- Voter registration office
- Any type of medical, behavioral health, or alternative medicine providers' offices
- Public assistance agencies, such as income support or food assistance

TIP

Many folks delay or even avoid applying for a legal name change for fear of the fees. Don't let this hold you back! Many courts include applications for free process or a fee waiver in the name change paperwork packet. Even if you have a job, fill these forms out and see if you qualify. Some national and local organizations work to help people who don't qualify for a fee waiver. One national organization that provides financial assistance is Trans Lifeline (go to `https://translife line.org/microgrants/#types`). See Chapter 12 for more help finding resources.

Getting your new state ID

Having a driver's license or state ID can make many things simpler now and in unexpected ways. You may have to show your ID to enroll in school, take a domestic flight, or start a new job. The U.S. government even has created standards for state-issued driver's licenses and ID cards that allow them to be considered secure and federally accepted forms of identification as well; these are called REAL IDs.

The X gender marker is a modern bureaucratic (or legal) way to recognize genders outside the binary. Most people grew up with the typical male (M) and female (F) gender markers; X is being introduced all over the world to provide an alternative. *Intersex* people (people whose bodies don't meet the typical definition of male or female) and non-binary people pushed for the X designation, but binary people can also use X to effectively decline to list their gender on documents.

The Movement Advancement Project (MAP) maintains an up-to-date map and web page detailing the ID laws and policies of each state, including which states are currently providing X gender markers on their IDs (`https://www.lgbtmap.org/equality-maps/identity_documents`). Figure 5-1 shows MAP's 2024 information about state ID changes.

If you live in one of the states that has created positive paths to getting an ID that matches your name and gender, you should be able to find the forms and instructions on your state's motor vehicle services website. Not only is the process different from state to state, but the state you live in determines whether you call that agency the DDS, BMV, DMV, or OMV.

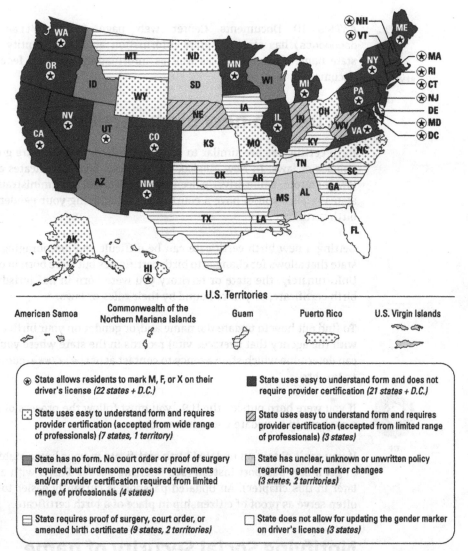

U.S. Territories

American Samoa   Commonwealth of the Northern Mariana Islands   Guam   Puerto Rico   U.S. Virgin Islands

⊛ State allows residents to mark M, F, or X on their driver's license *(22 states + D.C.)*

■ State uses easy to understand form and does not require provider certification *(21 states + D.C.)*

State uses easy to understand form and requires provider certification (accepted from wide range of professionals) *(7 states, 1 territory)*

State uses easy to understand form and requires provider certification (accepted from limited range of professionals) *(3 states)*

State has no form. No court order or proof of surgery required, but burdensome process requirements and/or provider certification required from limited range of professionals *(4 states)*

State has unclear, unknown or unwritten policy regarding gender marker changes *(3 states, 2 territories)*

State requires proof of surgery, court order, or amended birth certificate *(9 states, 2 territories)*

State does not allow for updating the gender marker on driver's license *(3 states)*

FIGURE 5-1: The Movement Advancement Project's 2024 state ID map.

TIP

If you live in one of the states that has made it harder to update your name and gender on your ID or simply doesn't allow transgender and non-binary people to change their documents, we know that's incredibly limiting and frustrating. You may consider joining the advocacy efforts in your location. We've been deeply involved in helping to change policies and laws (even the law that governs how you update the gender on your birth certificate) in our state, and we know transgender and non-binary people around the country are changing things and opening access for each other.

A4TE's ID Documents Center web page (https://transequality.org/documents) has state-by-state information about all identity documents and state name change laws, as well as information about all federal records and documents.

Securing a new birth certificate

Birth certificates are similar to state ID cards in that they are governed by state policies or laws. In New Mexico, for example, birth certificates are regulated by law or statute, while driver's licenses are governed by administrative policy. Some states require you to have a court order recognizing your gender to update your birth certificate.

Getting a new birth certificate can be difficult and discouraging if you live in a state that allows for changes to birth certificates but were born in one that doesn't. Unfortunately, the state or territory you were born in has jurisdiction over your birth certificate, so you're bound by their rules or laws.

To find out how to update the name and/or gender on your birth certificate, check with the agency that oversees vital records in the state where you were born. You can determine which state agency to contact at https://www.cdc.gov/nchs/w2w/index.htm.

If you were born outside the U.S., you must follow the process of the country you were born in to update your birth record.

If you can't obtain an updated birth certificate in your home state, you may want to get a new passport instead (see "Getting Set for Travel with a New Passport" later in this chapter). An updated passport is currently easier to obtain and can often serve as proof of citizenship in place of a birth certificate.

Notifying Social Security of name and gender changes

At the time we wrote this book, the Social Security Administration (SSA) has one of the easiest processes for changing your gender marker if you want M or F on your record. You simply submit an SS-5 form (application for a Social Security card); you don't need a medical provider to sign off on the change or any supporting documentation to verify your gender.

Your gender selection on the application doesn't have to match the sex or gender marker on any of your other documents, even the ones you submit as proof of identity with the SS-5. Acceptable forms of proof of identity include

>> U.S. driver's license

>> State-issued ID card

>> U.S. passport

Some people may want to change only their name and not their gender, or vice versa. You can do one or the other, or both, with the SS-5 form. If you're changing your name, you also need to submit a copy of your official name change court order. You should be aware that changes to your SSA records can trickle down to other databases you're listed in.

For more information, you can consult the SSA section linked to A4TE's ID Documents Center (https://transequality.org/documents/know-your-rights-social-security) or the frequently asked questions on the official SSA website (https://faq.ssa.gov/en-us/Topic/article/KA-01453).

REMEMBER

Although they don't currently have an X gender marker or any option for non-binary gender, the SSA indicates that they're looking into these options for the future.

Getting Set for Travel with a New Passport

A U.S. passport is often described as your ticket to travel outside the United States. It serves as a request to governments abroad to allow you to travel within their borders and grants you access to U.S. consular services while you're away from home. Having a valid passport opens up international opportunities for study, work, or even romance.

Beyond these benefits, a passport is also a fundamental government-issued REAL ID (a secure form of identification accepted by the U.S. government). You can use it as proof of identity and proof of citizenship in most situations, including to board domestic flights. So, having a valid passport can be a great solution if you live in a state that doesn't allow you to change your state ID or were born in a state that doesn't allow you to change your birth certificate.

In June 2021 the U.S. State Department moved to full *self-attestation* (the process of allowing an applicant to verify their document for themself) for gender changes on passports. This means you don't need a special letter from a medical or behavioral health provider or any other outside validation of your gender. You simply fill out and submit an application with your appropriate gender selected.

REMEMBER

At the beginning of 2022, X was added as a third gender option on the application for U.S. passports. The process of selecting X is exactly the same as it is for selecting M or F — you simply check the box.

WARNING

As of December 2024, many transgender organizations across the country are advising caution regarding obtaining new identity documents with an X gender marker. You can currently obtain a second passport if you have one with an X marker. You can find instructions here: https://travel.state.gov/content/travel/en/passports/have-passport/second-passport-book.html. Folks who already have an X on their passports and ID cards have to decide whether or not to hold on to them, and each person should choose what seems right for them. Many people are sticking with their X marker, for many different reasons, although there are some who feel safer having a binary gender marker at this time.

Modifying Military Records

WARNING

Even if you've never served in the military, this section may apply to you. In the U.S., people who were designated male at birth are required to register with the Selective Service System between the ages of 18 and 25, regardless of transition-related medical care or changes to gender markers on identity documents.

Registering with Selective Service

The Selective Service System was established in 1917 to manage the *draft* (mandatory enrollment for military service) by maintaining a database of eligible service members. In the U.S., men must register with the Selective Service and women are exempt, but this completely ignores the existence of transgender and non-binary citizens. Even in 2024, the regulations still require some groups of people to register while others are exempt.

The following people must register with the Selective Service:

>> All U.S. citizens who were designated male at birth and are 18 but not yet 26 years old

- » People who left active military service before the age of 26

- » People designated male at birth who were rejected for enlistment for any reason before age 26

- » Immigrants with permanent resident status

- » Undocumented immigrants

People who were designated female at birth are not required to register with the Selective Service. This requirement doesn't hinge on your current gender designation or any transition steps you have — or haven't — taken. However, if you apply for federal loans or grants as a transgender man, you may be asked for a Status Information Letter (SIL) to prove that you're exempt. You can apply for and download this letter online at the Selective Service's website (https://www.sss.gov/verify/). The SIL doesn't list the specific reason for your exemption, so it shouldn't out you on its own.

Updating other military records

On April 30, 2021, the U.S. Department of Defense (DOD) updated their policy on transgender military service to state that no person, based solely on their gender identity, will be

- » Involuntarily separated or discharged from military service

- » Denied reenlistment or continuation of military service

- » Subjected to adverse action or mistreatment

The process of transition during military service requires a medical diagnosis. According to the DOD policy:

> Gender transition begins when a Service member receives a diagnosis from a military medical provider indicating that gender transition is medically necessary, and then completes the medical care identified or approved by a military mental health or medical provider in a documented treatment plan as necessary to achieve stability in the self-identified gender. It concludes when the Service member's gender marker in [the Defense Enrollment Eligibility Reporting System (DEERS)] is changed and the Service member is recognized in [their] self-identified gender. Care and treatment may still be received after the gender marker is changed in DEERS . . ., but at that point, the Service member must meet all applicable military standards in the self-identified gender. With regard to facilities subject to regulation by the military, a Service member whose gender marker has been changed in DEERS will use those berthing, bathroom, and shower facilities associated with [their] gender marker in DEERS.

You can find the policy covering transition during military service online (https://www.esd.whs.mil/Portals/54/Documents/DD/issuances/dodi/130028p.pdf).

The U.S. Department of Veterans Affairs (VA) requires that transgender veterans be treated with safety, dignity, and respect and have access to care that's affirming and inclusive. The Veterans Health Administration (VHA) has added a new field to their database labeled Self-Identified Gender Identity (SIGI), which is distinct from the field labeled Birth Sex. Although you can update your birth sex through the VA privacy officer at your local facility, the VHA recommends that you just update your SIGI and keep the sex listed on your original birth certificate as your birth sex. You can update your SIGI (and your preferred name) at VA.gov.

If you have legally changed your name and want to update your name on your VA records, you must complete a form with your VA facility's privacy officer. This form has to be supported by at least one of the following unexpired official documents:

» State-issued driver's license with photo

» Passport with photo

» Federal, state, or local government-issued ID with photo, name, and date of birth

» Social Security card (along with an unexpired government-issued photo ID that includes either the old or the new name)

» Court order for name change (along with an unexpired government-issued photo ID that includes either the old or the new name)

For more information, check out the frequently asked questions on the VA's website (https://www.patientcare.va.gov/LGBT/Questions.asp).

Altering Immigration Documents

U.S. Citizenship and Immigration Services (USCIS) updated and streamlined the process for changing gender markers on most forms and documents on March 31, 2023. As of that date, updates to your gender are based on self-attestation. This means that you don't need any supporting documentation to validate your gender, and the gender you designate doesn't have to match the gender on any other supporting documentation you provide. For complete information, refer to the USCIS web page that explains how to update your documents (https://www.uscis.gov/tools/uscis-tools-and-resources/information-about-your-immigration-document/updating-or-correcting-your-documents).

WARNING

The significant exception to self-attestation for gender updates is Form N-565, Application for Replacement Naturalization/Citizenship Document (https://www.uscis.gov/sites/default/files/document/forms/n-565.pdf). This form requires supporting documentation for a gender change, such as a court order or a government-issued ID reflecting the gender change.

To change your name on your immigration records, you need to provide documentation of your new legal name (most likely, your court order). Go to the web page listed in the first paragraph of this section to update your personal information with USCIS.

Chapter **6**

Planning for the Future

Planning for the future is a huge topic that could probably fill another book! What we mean by this chapter title is thinking about relationships and family, including plans around kids (or not), marriage, and doing the difficult work of preparing for your death. Everyone has to contemplate these big questions, but for transgender and non-binary people there are some special considerations. You may not have the support of your original family, for example, which means specifying your wishes, or making sure that you have legally adopted your kids, can ensure that you are protected.

In this chapter, you find guidance for considering what kinds of relationships you want to be in, and your vision of family. You also get important information about a topic that can be hard to talk and think about: organizing your medical and financial affairs. Considering these aspects of the future, especially strategizing about end-of-life plans or advance directives if you become sick or incapacitated, isn't exactly fun. But it *is* important.

WARNING

A critical fact to remember about the legal documents discussed in this chapter is that they vary from state to state. It's extremely important to research the documents for your state and how to execute them in order to ensure that your plans are locked in.

Doing Your Advance Planning

There is no smooth way to move from having your kids to planning for death or future illness or injury. But it's all part of the full circle of our lifetimes, and it all needs to be addressed. While straight and *cisgender* folks (people whose gender and sex match up) can and do avoid long-term planning, some transgender and non-binary people have reported feeling more intimidated about everything from family planning to wills and advance directives. If you feel scared about making plans for your future, or even just a little confused, read on! We hope you're more informed and confident about these vital steps by the end of the chapter.

We explore a few basic documents in this chapter. As you read through it, you discover more about

>> Wills

>> Power of attorney forms

>> Advance directives

>> Nonprobate transfers

The following sections delve into each of these topics.

Understanding wills and why they're important

Many folks feel like they don't need a will if they don't have a lot of assets, don't own property, or aren't parents or guardians. However, it's important for everyone to have a will. After you die, decisions and arrangements must be made. This is true even if you preplan your funeral and the disposition of your body (for example, burial or cremation). So, at a minimum, you need a will to appoint the person you want to take on this role when you're gone. The person who settles your estate is often called an *executor* but is sometimes referred to as a *personal representative*.

Your executor will file your death certificate and will with the probate court, and if no one contests (challenges) the will, the court will officially name the executor as your estate's representative. This allows financial and medical institutions, your employer, banks, insurance companies, funeral homes, and other entities to recognize their authority to act on behalf of your estate. Some of the executor's jobs include the following:

>> Overseeing funeral arrangements and disposition of your body

>> Taking inventory of any assets or debts attributed to your estate

>> Settling debts

>> Distributing any assets to beneficiaries according to your will

If someone comes forward and contests your will, settling your estate after your death can become complicated. However, if nobody contests your will, probating it should be straightforward and relatively simple.

Many courts have probate forms, including wills, on their websites. Self-help guides and even self-help desks are also commonly available through the courts. Some nonprofit organizations provide free clinics and even hotlines and websites that offer assistance with the process. Search online to find local resources in your state.

TIP

If you have a hard time finding local options, the American Bar Association has a web page that focuses on finding free legal help (https://www.americanbar.org/groups/legal_services/flh-home/flh-free-legal-help/). Some websites offer basic wills you can fill out for free or for a minimal fee (up to $100). FreeWill is one reputable free website you may find helpful (https://www.freewill.com/about).

Because wills are governed by state law, the requirements and forms vary widely for each state. Some of the rules are definitely not logical. For instance, in New York state, someone making a copy of your will isn't allowed to remove the staples before copying it. If they do take out the staples without submitting a notarized form to the court explaining the reason and promising that no changes were made, the whole will may be invalid.

Most states require a valid will to have the following components:

>> **Your full legal name:** This is another great example of why it can be life changing to legally change your name. Your will has to be completed with whatever legal name you have at that time.

>> **A statement that you are of sound mind:** Each state has its own requirements around this, but there is often language within the will itself, stating "I, (your name), being of sound mind and body . . ." This can be validated by medical professionals but sometimes is attested to by the presence of the required witnesses to the signing.

>> **Two choices for executor/personal representative:** You need to name your first choice and one backup pick in case your first choice isn't available for any reason when the time comes.

>> **A list of people you're leaving your estate to:** The division of assets is often specified by percentage, but not always. For example, you may leave 100 percent of your assets to a partner, child, or close friend. Or, you may split your estate equally between a group of friends and/or relatives. It's just important to make sure that your percentages add up to 100 percent.

>> **Your signature:** You have to sign your will in front of two witnesses. Typically, it's best to have your signature certified by a *notary public* (a state-appointed official who serves as an impartial witness to the signing of documents and establishes the authenticity of the signatures).

TIP

All banks have a notary on-site and they will notarize your signature for a small fee, usually around $10. If you go to your own bank, it is usually a free service.

Designating a power of attorney

In addition to a will, you should consider designating a *power of attorney* (POA), or giving someone the authority to act and make decisions on your behalf. Just as with wills, the rules and requirements vary from state to state, but a POA is accepted in all states.

A POA can be *durable*, meaning it doesn't expire if you become unable to communicate, or *nondurable*, meaning it's assigned for a limited time and purpose. For example, you can execute a nondurable POA if you're going on an extended trip out of the country and need to designate someone to conduct financial business for you while you're gone. There are many valid uses for nondurable POAs, but they're not the type of POA used for advance planning. A durable POA means that the authority of the person you designate does not expire if you become unable to communicate.

Many courts will presume that a POA is durable unless it states otherwise. However, it's a good idea to explicitly state that you are executing a durable POA just to ward off any misunderstandings during what can be a difficult and confusing time — for example, if you are hospitalized after a car accident.

There are three types of POAs:

>> **General:** This POA gives your agent the power to act on your behalf in all situations as if they were legally you.

>> **Financial:** This is one of the limited POAs. It allows your agent to act on your behalf in financial matters that you specify. You can empower your financial POA to make deposits and withdrawals from your account, but not file your taxes, for example.

>> **Medical:** Medical POAs are also limited. With a medical POA, you authorize your agent to make decisions about your healthcare, such as whether to allow medical professionals to perform surgery or insert a feeding tube.

You don't have to designate the same person to have medical and financial decision-making power for you. You may have folks in your life you trust to do one or the other. It's a great idea to think about who you feel safe and comfortable giving control over important aspects of your life and well-being. You should have a backup selected for your POA in case the primary person is unable to do the job at the time.

POAs are especially important for folks who aren't married. Legal marriage confers the power to make medical and financial decisions onto your spouse. If you're partnered and not married, it's very important to execute a POA so that your partner is respected as your agent if needed.

A final important consideration is that your POA, especially in the medical role, must be able to put aside their feelings about not only approving various medical procedures and interventions, but also about allowing you not to be resuscitated if that's your written wish. This isn't an easy ask of people who love you a lot.

If you don't have someone in your life who seems like a good fit for this job, you can appoint a professional, like an attorney. You can also accomplish some of the medical decision-making by creating an advance directive (see the next section) and addressing as many possibilities as you can in that document.

TIP

Each trans and non-binary person is different. Some people have great relationships with their *family of origin* (the family you were born into, adopted into, or grew up with). Others, however, have complicated or even antagonistic relationships with these relatives. There have been many accounts of transgender people being buried in clothing of the wrong gender, having memorial services that referred to them using only their *deadname* (the name you were given at birth but no longer use), or having their gender-affirming care taken away when they were unable to communicate for themselves. This underlines why it's crucial to take charge by executing whatever combination of wills, advance directives, POAs, and PODs makes sense for you and making your own decisions ahead of time.

Making advance directives

An *advance directive*, also known as a *living will*, is a legal document that lays out your wishes about your medical care if you're unable to communicate for yourself. Some of the important topics that can be addressed in an advance directive include

>> **Pain relief:** You may want to specify whether you want all available pain relief options, or whether you have limits on what you want. Some people opt out of pain relief options that can prolong their life in certain circumstances.

>> **Life-sustaining options:** A host of medical treatments and interventions, such as CPR, mechanical ventilation, artificial nutrition and hydration, dialysis, and antibiotics, are available these days. In your advance directive, you can specify which ones you want and don't want, as well as when you'd like treatments to stop if you aren't getting better.

>> **Removal from life support:** An advance directive allows you to specify when you want to be removed from life support systems. For some people brain death is the threshold, while others want all possible measures taken until their heart stops beating.

>> **Tissue, organ, brain, and body donation:** Researching and deciding ahead of time to donate your body or brain to science, or donate your organs and tissues to people who need them, is a great idea. Whether or not this is for you, an advance directive is a chance to think meaningfully about the incredible difference this gift can make, and specify your wishes in advance.

WARNING

After all the planning and work you put into it, you may be wondering what happens if your advance directive isn't followed. Even though these documents are legally recognized, some situations aren't covered by a living will. Complex medical issues that your advance directive doesn't address can arise, and some medical providers have refused the wishes outlined in a living will. If something in your advance directive violates the policy of the healthcare institution or currently accepted healthcare standards, for example, a provider may be unable to carry out your wishes. Some medical providers have refused to follow advance directives because the patient's wishes violate their conscience. If this occurs, the provider is expected to inform your representative immediately and consider transferring your care to another provider.

You can even specify things like how are you treated and housed in nursing facilities. People have been forced into rooming situations with people who do not match their gender without a strong advocate and/or an advance directive. This is your chance to say what you want and how you want to be treated. Nobody has ever had their wishes respected when they weren't even expressed! As we say earlier, the law of your state and the policies of the institutions can still create a situation where your wishes are not followed, but this can be your best opportunity to try to protect your future self.

TIP

It's important to consider the pros and cons of a POA versus an advance directive if your state separates them. Although many decisions can be addressed in an advance directive, a POA is more flexible if situations that you didn't anticipate arise. That's why you have to have a lot of trust in your POA. An advance directive is always exactly what you specified, in your own voice. Because POAs and advance directives are meant to cover many of the same concerns, some states, like California, use the terminology *advance healthcare directive* for a combined living will and medical POA.

Setting up nonprobate transfers

Nonprobate assets aren't required to pass through probate after your death. In other words, a judge doesn't have to rule on them. Earlier in this chapter we describe what happens when your executor takes your will to court and probates it (see "Understanding wills and why they're important"). Nonprobate assets can be distributed before probate takes place. Nonprobate transfers are not part of the probate process, and the executor does not distribute them. Instead, the bank or the insurance company or a county clerk makes the transfer of ownership to a person you designated while you were alive.

REMEMBER

As with other estate planning, it's important to remember that laws are different in each state, so as you set up your arrangements for nonprobate transfers, use the internet and local legal resources to be sure you're in compliance with the laws and rules where you live.

Having said that, every bank should allow you to designate a payable on death (POD) beneficiary for your checking, savings, certificate of deposit, individual retirement, money market, or investment accounts. Some banks even allow you to complete a form online specifying who your POD beneficiary is. If you can't do it online, you can go to your bank and fill out a signature card to be placed on file. You can have more than one POD beneficiary, but make sure the percentage you leave to each beneficiary totals 100%. If you designate a POD beneficiary on your bank account, remember that that account will not be available to your executor to distribute in accordance with your will. This is because upon your death, the assets in the bank account became the property of the person you designated, meaning it belongs to that person and is not part of your estate.

At the time this book went to press, 27 states and D.C. offer what are called *transfer on death* (TOD) deeds. A TOD deed is a legal document you file to designate who should receive specific real property at the time of your death without passing through probate. Instead, the county clerk updates the warranty deed based on the TOD.

You may have a retirement account at work that you've forgotten about, or a life insurance policy through your job that you aren't even aware of. If you're employed, double-check with your employer about these things. If you have either type of account, designate a beneficiary or multiple beneficiaries.

Again, these are all called nonprobate transfers because a judge does not have to rule on them. As long as the designated person or people have a death certificate, that is all that is typically needed to get the ball rolling on moving these assets.

A final nonprobate asset to consider is taking out a small life insurance policy on yourself for the benefit of your executor or personal representative. Many factors affect the price of an individual policy, but even at age 55, a person in reasonably good health may pay $20 or less per month for a $10,000 policy. Making your executor the beneficiary on this policy would quickly free up funds to cover any unexpected expenses related to your after-death arrangements. Even if you prepay for the bulk of the expenses, other things will crop up. The check is often issued within a week or two of your death, so your executor is relieved of any worries about having to cover anything themself.

As we make clear in this chapter, being someone's executor isn't an easy job. It can be rewarding and an honor to help someone you love in this way. But it's often thankless work, too. So, if anything is left over from your life insurance policy after your funeral and other expenses are covered, the remaining funds can be a small gesture of thanks to your executor.

Safeguarding Your Important Documents

After you've decided on your executor, one important step you don't want to skip is telling them! The person you've selected should know that they have been named in your will to act in this capacity. Once they've accepted the job, and all your documents have been fully executed with notarized signatures, you should give the executor a copy of them. If your executor is in a stable, safe living situation, you can even consider giving them the originals for safekeeping.

WARNING

After your death, when these documents become vitally important, the only ones that will matter are the original signed versions. Distributing copies to key people isn't a bad idea; that way, those people know what you want and can assist in carrying out your wishes. However, the courts will not accept copies of your will and other estate-related documents under any circumstances. Hiding these documents or storing them in a safe deposit box without telling anyone so that nobody can find them after your death would be a tragic mistake.

If you have a stable living situation, store your will and related documents with your other important papers. An attorney who helped you prepare these documents will often keep the originals for you as a courtesy. Just be sure your representatives and beneficiaries know where they are.

REMEMBER, TAKE YOUR TIME

As you can see, you have a lot to think about when it comes to planning for the future. Whether you're weighing advance medical or financial planning, or if or how to have a family, it's important to take the time to really consider and get in touch with your values and what matters to you. If you make these important decisions from that place, hopefully they'll be decisions you can feel good about!

Don't forget that there's help out there if you need it. Numerous websites offer assistance with wills and other advance planning, and you can research local and state resources online, too. Various nonprofit organizations provide legal assistance to low-income folks, and some LGBTQ centers have legal clinics that can help with estate and family planning. Many of the Planned Parenthood affiliates around the country are knowledgeable and culturally fluent about transgender and non-binary patients, and can be valuable resources when it comes to family planning and even referrals for services like genetic tissue recovery and storage. Don't be afraid to reach out for help and information!

3
Navigating Medical Transition

IN THIS CHAPTER

» **Managing your preventive care**

» **Selecting healthcare providers**

» **Understanding evaluation for gender treatment**

» **Experiencing stress-related illness**

» **Maneuvering aesthetics and hygiene issues**

Chapter **7**

Considering Primary Healthcare

S electing healthcare providers for gender-affirming care is tough, especially if you live in an area without many trained clinicians and/or with legislative limitations on which treatments are available. But you have options even if you're in that situation.

In this chapter, you dive into the details of the medical aspects of transition for the first time. This is a huge topic that's covered in Chapters 7, 8, 9, 10, and 11. In this chapter, you explore primary healthcare, beginning with an overview of preventive healthcare for trans and non-binary people. We also give you guidance on choosing the healthcare provider(s) who will oversee your care.

Evaluations for gender-related treatments can be overwhelming, so this chapter outlines some of the different ways that type of appointment can go. And because transgender and non-binary people carry higher *allostatic loads* (the wear and tear on the body over time caused by repeated or chronic stress), we address stress-related illnesses, and touch on some ways to ease your stress and its effects on your health.

Finally, this chapter highlights some hygiene practices you may need to change or become familiar with if you're undergoing medical transition, allowing you to explore different aspects of aesthetics, from hair removal to facials. (*Aesthetics*, sometimes spelled *esthetics*, are cosmetic practices used for beautifying skin and hair.)

Taking Charge of Your Preventive Healthcare

Navigating healthcare can be tricky for anyone, but transgender and non-binary folks usually face a few extra challenges and considerations. Unfortunately, preventive healthcare for trans and non-binary people is just beginning to be studied seriously. That means the best information about how to manage your health before you develop an illness or chronic condition is somewhere in the future.

But some helpful guidelines are already apparent. One of the most basic, but important, is the concept that if you have a body part, your medical provider should follow the same healthcare guidelines they would follow for a *cisgender* person (whose gender and sex match up) with that body part. The following sections cover a few healthcare issues transgender and non-binary people may have concerns or questions about.

REMEMBER

It's totally within your rights to ask your healthcare provider to use gender-affirming or gender-neutral language, especially if they're referring to a part of your body that you have strong negative, or just complex, feelings about.

Starting off on the right foot

TIP

You shouldn't have to educate your healthcare provider in order to get the care you need, but a lot of trans and non-binary patients find themselves in that situation. Some resources you can share with your primary care provider include the following:

>> Guidelines on primary care from the University of California San Francisco's Center of Excellence for Transgender Health (https://transcare.ucsf.edu/guidelines)

>> Current standards of care for transgender healthcare from the World Professional Association for Transgender Health, or WPATH (https://www.wpath.org/soc8)

» A paper on gender-affirming care from the National Library of Medicine (https://www.ncbi.nlm.nih.gov/pmc/articles/PMC9341318/)

» A paper on caring for transgender and non-binary patients from the American Academy of Family Physicians (https://www.aafp.org/pubs/afp/issues/2018/1201/p645.html)

Recognizing potential risks of gender-affirming care

One element of your health you may have concerns about is your bone health. Specific transition factors, namely any combination of treatments that would cause you to have sustained hormone levels under what is typical, can put you at higher risk for low bone density, but the recommendation for trans and non-binary people is to start bone density screening at age 65. Screening can be considered between 50 and 64 if other bone health risk factors are present.

Right now, it's not completely clear whether people on hormone therapy are at higher risk for cardiovascular disease. So, if you're using hormones as part of your gender-affirming care, your screening for cardiovascular disease will be done according to the current recommendations for all people in your age group and with your risk factors. If you have concerns or questions, your healthcare provider can calculate your atherosclerotic cardiovascular disease (ASCVD) risk score. Just be aware that it may be more accurate to use your predominant sex hormone when selecting gender on the ASCVD risk calculator.

There's also no current information that indicates people on hormone therapy have higher rates of any type of cancer. If you have a particular body part or organ and you meet the criteria for cancer screening based on certain risk factors or symptoms, you should consider screening regardless of hormone use. For example, if you have breast tissue, the breast cancer screening guidelines for you would be the same ones used for cisgender women. Likewise, cervical cancer screening is recommended for anyone with a cervix, and guidelines used for cis women are appropriate regardless of hormone use.

Caring for your sexual health

A final important consideration regarding your preventive healthcare is sexual health and satisfaction. Some folks identify their orientation as *asexual*, meaning that they lack sexual feelings toward other people, or have a more general lack of desire for sexual activity. (Asexual people don't see their feelings about sex as pathological or lacking. They aren't necessarily repulsed by sex, and they may engage in sex occasionally and may have romantic feelings for others.) If you don't engage in sexual activity, for any reason, then you shouldn't need to be screened for sexually transmitted infections (STIs) or be concerned about pregnancy.

If you do engage in sexual behavior with others, you should follow the STI screening guidelines for all sexually active people supported by the U.S. Centers for Disease Control and Prevention (CDC) and the U.S. Preventive Services Task Force. If you meet the criteria for the preventive medication known as pre-exposure prophylaxis (PrEP) — that is, you are negative for HIV but at higher risk because of your sexual practices or injection drug use — it's a great idea to talk with your healthcare provider about taking PrEP. You may also want to have a look at *Safer Sex for Trans Bodies*, an amazing online resource about sexual health and trans people from the Human Rights Campaign (https://www.hrc.org/resources/safer-sex-for-trans-bodies).

REMEMBER

Talking about sex and sexual health can be hard, even with friends and partners. So, it makes sense that it can be difficult to bring these issues up with clinicians. Your sexual health and satisfaction are important and can be a big part of your life and overall health. A good healthcare provider will ask questions and focus on you and your needs in a discussion of sexual health and practices. Hopefully, you can be direct with your provider about the language you prefer, not just with regard to your chosen name and pronouns, but also when you're talking about your body. Some trans folks have special names for their genitals, like *joystick* or *front hole*. But your request can be as simple as asking a provider to say *chest* rather than *breasts* during your time together.

WARNING

A significant number of trans masculine people on testosterone therapy report pelvic pain, especially during sex. A recent paper notes the correlation and urges the healthcare community to do more research (https://www.ncbi.nlm.nih.gov/pmc/articles/PMC10079239/). Don't suffer in silence! Talk to your healthcare provider if you're having pain. It may be a sign of something more serious like *endometriosis* (abnormal uterine tissue growth outside the uterus), or your provider may be able to offer solutions to ease your pain.

Choosing Healthcare Providers

You may have many knowledgeable healthcare providers in your area, making your toughest decision finding the one who is the best fit for you. Or you may live in a place where finding someone who knows anything about transgender or non-binary patients is a real challenge. Either way, this section provides guidance to help you find a viable option to start or maintain whatever treatment you want or need as a trans or non-binary patient.

If you have a lot of choices, it's important to home in on some criteria you can use to figure out which healthcare provider is right for you. In general, here are some good ways to find medical providers and narrow down your options:

>> **Ask people you know.** In the transgender community, word of mouth has been the preferred, and sometimes only, way to find a doctor who knows about trans and non-binary patients and treats folks with respect and care. The best place to start is with people you already know and trust: your friends, family, and coworkers — and especially other trans and non-binary people.

>> **Check for a directory online.** You can also consult some good online directories. If you have a local organization like the Transgender Resource Center of New Mexico, they may have a structured directory (see the Provider Directory page at https://tgrcnm.org/providers), or at least be able to provide email or verbal referrals to local providers. If there isn't a similar organization in your area (or even if there is), you can check national online databases. At the time of writing, good directories can be found on the following websites:

- OutCare Health's OutList (https://www.outcarehealth.org/outlist/)

- WPATH's Provider Directory (https://www.wpath.org/provider/search)

- LGBTQ+ Healthcare Directory (https://lgbtqhealthcaredirectory.org/)

>> **Check your insurance (if you have it).** If you don't have health insurance, it's absolutely worth checking to see if you qualify for Medicaid in the state where you live. You can find out more about eligibility in your state on the Medicaid website (https://www.medicaid.gov/about-us/where-can-people-get-help-medicaid-chip/index.html). If you already have health insurance, look for healthcare providers who are in your network, because the care you get from in-network providers is much more likely to be covered by your policy.

>> **Consider logistics.** Do you have reliable transportation to get to a medical provider that isn't close to your home? Do you need to be able to use telehealth sometimes (or always)? Do you have to go to an outside lab or radiology group to get blood work or X-rays? If any of these considerations, or others, poses significant issues for you, now is a great time to find out what you need to know.

>> **Make sure the provider has the right knowledge.** This may or may not be knowledge specifically related to caring for trans people. Whatever you're planning to see a clinician for, it's a good idea to confirm that they have experience and expertise in that area of medicine. You can call the office to ask whether they've ever seen trans patients in their practice, what the bathrooms are like at the clinic or office, or anything else you want to know

ahead of your visit. Sometimes a clinician who doesn't have experience with trans medicine is open to learning, so the next point is really important.

>> **After your visit, reflect on the experience.** Did the provider listen to you and your concerns? Did they interrupt or condescend to you? Did they encourage you to ask questions? How much time did they spend with you? How were you treated by the other people you encountered at the office, including support or administrative staff?

REMEMBER

It's 100 percent okay — you really owe it to yourself — to find someone else to assist you if you feel disrespected or as if the provider or their staff didn't care about you or treated you poorly in any way.

TIP

If there's no healthcare provider in your area who offers transition care, you can now get care from some online providers. Some provide primary care and mental health services, and some take insurance. At the time of writing some options are

>> Circle Medical (https://www.circlemedical.com/what-we-treat/hormone-therapy)

>> QueerMed (https://queermed.com)

>> FOLX (https://www.folxhealth.com)

>> Plume (https://getplume.co)

Understanding Gender Dysphoria Evaluations

Although there's currently plenty of debate among insurers about whether to require a diagnosis of gender dysphoria before covering healthcare costs, many insurance plans in the United States do require a diagnosis of gender dysphoria before they cover gender-related medical expenses and behavioral healthcare. *Gender dysphoria*, a diagnosis in the American Psychiatric Association's Diagnostic and Statistical Manual of Mental Disorders, 5th edition (DSM-5), is a persistent, consistent knowledge, lasting 6 months or longer, that your gender doesn't match your designated sex at birth. Elements of gender dysphoria include an incompatibility between your experienced gender and your primary and/or secondary sex characteristics, a desire to align your primary and secondary sex characteristics with your experienced gender, and a desire to be viewed and treated by others as your experienced gender.

You have to research your insurance plan to find out if it requires a diagnosis of gender dysphoria. Not every healthcare provider will feel capable or willing to provide this diagnosis, but any clinician trained and licensed to manage behavioral health can diagnose gender dysphoria. This covers counselors and therapists but also includes medical providers.

WARNING

Some folks who have the financial means opt to pay for their treatment out of pocket, rather than have a gender dysphoria diagnosis in their chart. Your medical and behavioral health records can be *subpoenaed* (summoned into a court proceeding with an official document called *a writ of subpoena*). You have to decide whether you're comfortable with official records documenting your gender status, and with leaving those records behind when you're gone.

REMEMBER

You do *not* have to experience gender dysphoria to be transgender or non-binary. You also don't have to experience gender dysphoria to want or need various forms of medical transition. The diagnostic code can impact your ability to utilize your insurance to pay for treatment, but it's not at all a prerequisite to being trans.

Who can evaluate and provide care for you?

The best-case scenario is that your gender care will be provided in a team-based setting consisting of primary care, endocrinology, nursing, behavioral health, and case management. However, we know this type of care isn't always accessible. Some cases may call for a referral to a specialist, but most patients' issues can be addressed by a primary care provider.

Increasingly, primary care is recognized as the most appropriate venue for trans and non-binary patients to receive hormone therapy and coordinate any other treatment goals. The best primary care providers are

>> **Patient-centered:** They recognize that everyone's gender journey is different, and that there's no "full transition" that has a shared meaning, and they follow the patient's lead in terms of personal gender goals, which may not include medications or surgery.

>> **Trauma-informed:** They take a healing-centered approach based on creating a safe environment where patient empowerment and dignity is supported, and on recognizing people's inherent strengths and capabilities.

These qualities show up in details like inclusive intake forms and bathrooms, as well as patients' personal experience with the provider. It's important for the practice to create a clinical environment that's affirming by, for example, having intake forms with gender-neutral language and inclusive options for gender selection. All clinic staff should be trained on the importance of using each patient's correct name and pronouns, and on the significance of introducing themselves with their own pronouns during appointments.

What do evaluations involve?

At your first visit, a healthcare professional may ask about your history, including your gender, gender journey, social support, past medical/surgical/behavioral health history, family history, current behavioral health counseling, and goals for coming to see them. Your care goals may include primary care, hormone therapy, and/or gender-confirmation surgeries. There's no single or "correct" way to chart your gender journey, and the best clinicians will follow your lead and support and assist you in reaching your goals.

Your healthcare provider should use your name, gender (as stated by you), and pronouns throughout the visit and consistently in their documentation. An example of an *identification statement* (how you are noted in your medical chart) may read "25-year-old male (designated female at birth, or DFAB, he/him) here to discuss hypertension."

Current standards of care encourage medical providers to engage in a practice known as *informed consent* (a process in which the provider explains the treatment being proposed, the risks, the benefits, and any options other than the primary one being considered). The provider also assesses the patient's ability to provide consent, their understanding of the information provided, and any factors that may influence their decision, and then, together, they proceed with treatment.

WARNING

A lot of folks have had bad experiences with medical providers or in clinical settings. Some of these experiences have even involved inappropriate physical exams that don't align with the patient's reason for seeking care. While trauma responses can make you freeze up or want to run away, you always have the right to say no to any physical exam or treatment and to ask for someone else to be in the room with you. If possible, bringing an advocate to your appointments, someone you really trust and can be vulnerable in front of, can make a huge difference as well. You can discuss your boundaries and wishes with this person and ask them to help protect you during the exam. Also, if your provider requires a letter from a behavioral health provider before initiating hormone treatment, that may be a yellow flag, because a medical provider should be able to provide this diagnosis without outside assistance, just as they would with diabetes.

Examining Stress-Related Illness

Many Americans are familiar with the idea that a high level of stress can contribute to physical and medical challenges. For example, a stressed-out person having a heart attack has been used as a plot device in many plays, TV shows, and movies. But in the 1990s, a small number of clinicians started putting the pieces together to see that stressful events happening to kids under 18 (adverse childhood experiences, or ACEs) continue to cause far-reaching health issues in adulthood like pregnancy complications, cancer, diabetes, and increased risk of experiencing sexual violence. For adults, the financial burden of health conditions that are associated with ACEs is 14 trillion dollars per year in the United States alone (https://pmc.ncbi.nlm.nih.gov/articles/PMC10701608/).

You may be wondering what stress-related illness has to do with being transgender or non-binary. Many people who carry minority characteristics experience stress-related illness, and the prevalence of stress-related conditions across trans populations backs that up. Unfortunately, trans and non-binary folks appear to have higher rates of conditions like depression, anxiety, self-harm, suicidal thoughts and attempts, and substance use in addition to autoimmune issues (including mast cell activation), autonomic nervous system dysregulation (such as postural orthostatic tachycardia syndrome), chronic pain, metabolic disorders, and cardiovascular concerns.

Recognizing your own resilience is one way to navigate this difficult reality; maintaining connections to other people is another. And figuring out how to advocate for yourself and be in the driver's seat of your preventive healthcare and wellness is a big step in trying to avoid poor health outcomes.

REMEMBER

When you have trauma, it can be very hard to advocate for yourself, so nothing in this section is meant to make you feel bad if you find that impossible right now. We hope to offer you some tools for building the confidence to seek the care you need.

Acknowledging structural determinants of health

From 1995 to 1997, healthcare giant Kaiser Permanente conducted a study in Southern California that tied child abuse and neglect and other family trauma to poor physical and mental health in adulthood (you can find out more online at https://www.cdc.gov/violenceprevention/aces/about.html). The Kaiser study labeled these stressful events that happen to kids under 18 *adverse childhood experiences* (ACEs).

For the purposes of this study, three types of ACEs were outlined: abuse, neglect, and household dysfunction. Abuse includes physical, emotional, or sexual incidents. Both physical and emotional neglect are considered. Household dysfunction encompassed issues such as mental illness, a relative who is incarcerated, domestic violence, divorce, and substance abuse. The prevalence for ACEs was variable, but significant among the 17,000 respondents:

>> Emotional abuse — 10.6%

>> Sexual abuse — 20.7%

>> Physical abuse — 28.3%

>> Physical neglect — 9.9%

>> Emotional neglect — 14.8%

>> Incarcerated household member — 4.7%

>> Mother treated violently — 12.7%

>> Household mental illness — 19.4%

>> Parental divorce — 23.3%

>> Household substance abuse — 26.9%

There is much more information about the ACE study and the growing body of knowledge online. One starting place to check out is https://www.cdc.gov/aces/about/index.html.

The understanding of how childhood trauma affects adult health has been expanded by the writing and scholarship of people like Gabor Maté and Bessel van der Kolk, who ground childhood trauma in the experience of not being seen or heard. According to the research conducted by these scientists and others, when children don't have attachment and attunement from their caregivers and significant adults in their lives, their brains are set up not just for compulsive behaviors (sometimes called addiction) but also for many of the illnesses that are rooted in stress and trauma.

When you think about it, you start to realize that mainstream U.S. culture doesn't really prioritize attachment and attunement between parents and babies and kids. For example, the United States doesn't compare well to other countries around the world that provide a significant amount of parental leave when a child is born or adopted. And many other types of support offered to new parents in other countries (such as postpartum pelvic floor therapy for new parents in France, or family leave that lasts up to 24 weeks in Denmark, giving parents and babies the opportunity to bond) haven't been introduced in the United States. In other words, individual parents aren't necessarily to blame for this type of very common childhood trauma, because a lot of the attachment and attunement issues are structural and rooted in a society's priorities.

So, U.S. culture already creates a lot of barriers to achieving good health. Now, factor in being a trans or non-binary or gender-variant kid on top of that. Many of these young people — even those who know they are loved by their families — can't shake the feeling of being different. As LGBTQ kids grow up, they often report feeling somewhat outside their family of origin, and a lot of folks in these communities talk about *chosen family*, meaning the people you form close relationships with, lean on in times of trouble, and can really be yourself with. Seeking out and cultivating human connection is definitely one of the antidotes to some of these stress-related health risks.

TECHNICAL
STUFF

The 2015 U.S. Transgender Survey, with nearly 28,000 trans and non-binary respondents, found that almost 60 percent of respondents reported significant rejection from their family of origin because of their gender identity, and almost one-sixth reported harassment so severe that they left school (in either K-12 or higher education settings). Additionally, 19 percent were refused medical care because of their gender, and 41 percent reported attempting suicide (compared with 1.6 percent of the general population). It is crucial to remember that these outcomes aren't rooted in the simple fact of someone's transgender or non-binary identities. You should not be afraid that just being transgender puts you at risk for self-harm or addiction. The way that other people treat trans folks, and the stigma, discrimination and even violence that some people experience, are at the bottom of these statistics.

REMEMBER

Increasingly, loneliness, isolation, and disconnection are being studied as social determinants of health. Books like Johann Hari's *Lost Connections* and *Together* by Vivek Murthy (the 19th and 21st U.S. Surgeon General) provide in-depth explorations of the many ways that loneliness and disconnection are causing negative physical and behavioral health outcomes in people. In fact, Murthy illustrates that loneliness can be as deadly for humans as smoking cigarettes!

So, whether trauma is developmental, whether it's chronic or acute, or whether it occurs in childhood or adulthood, its impact on mental and physical health is finally being acknowledged. Some stress-related health issues now associated with trauma include

>> Chronic shame

>> Tendency to reenact dangerous situations

>> Loss of fundamental sense of safety

>> Changes in brain architecture

>> Reactive immune system

>> Damage from prolonged exposure to stress hormones

>> Changes to telomeres at cellular level (big words for what amounts to premature aging and degeneration of the cells)

Figure 7-1, from the ECHO Training Institute, lays out some of these impacts of trauma. Their infographic at http://echotraining.org/ provides more detail about each of these impacts:

>> Re-enactment: Recreating the childhood dynamic expecting the same result but hoping for a different one. This strategy is doomed to failure because the need is in the past and cannot be resolved. Also, you will interpret anything as confirmation that you have been betrayed once more.

>> Loss of safety: The world becomes a place where anything can happen.

>> Loss of danger cues: How do you know what is dangerous when someone you trust hurts you and this is then your "normal"?

>> Loss of trust: This is especially true if the abuser is a family member or a close family friend.

>> Shame: Huge, overwhelming, debilitating shame. As a child, even getting an exercise wrong at school can trigger the shame. The child may grow into an adult who cannot bear to be in the wrong because it is such a trigger.

>> Loss of intimacy: For survivors of sexual abuse, sexual relationships can either become something to avoid or are entered into for approval (since the child learns that sex is a way to get the attention they crave) and the person may be labeled "promiscuous."

>> Dissociation: Often, to cope with what is happening to the body during the abuse, the child will dissociate (disconnect the consciousness from what is happening). Later, this becomes a coping strategy that is used whenever the survivor is feeling overwhelmed.

>> Loss of physical connection to the body: Survivors of sexual and physical abuse often have a hard time being in their body. This disconnection from the body makes some therapies known to aid trauma recovery, such as yoga, harder for these survivors.

>> Loss of sense of self: One of the roles of the primary caregiver is to help us discover our identity by reflecting who we are back to us. If the abuser was a parent or caregiver, then that sense of self is not well developed and can leave us feeling phony or fake.

>> Loss of self-worth: Trauma survivors can swing between feeling special, with grandiose beliefs about themselves, and feeling dirty and "bad." This self-aggrandizement is an elaborate defense against the unbearable feeling of being an outcast and unworthy of love.

TIP

If you recognize any of this in yourself, it may feel rough. Once again, know that you are not alone. There are ways to address trauma, and understanding the causes and effects is a huge first step.

REMEMBER

Trauma is one important determinant of health, but it's vital to remember the role of systemic or structural determinants of health as well. Various health experts and organizations define these in many different ways, but the CDC emphasizes these five structural determinants of health:

>> Healthcare access and quality

>> Education access and quality

>> Social and community context

>> Economic stability

>> Neighborhood and built environment (man-made spaces in a community)

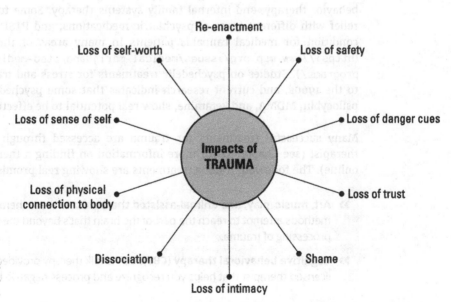

FIGURE 7-1:
Health impacts
of trauma.

Re-enactment

Loss of self-worth

Loss of safety

Loss of sense of self

Loss of danger cues

Impacts of TRAUMA

Loss of physical connection to body

Loss of trust

Dissociation

Shame

Loss of intimacy

Managing trauma for trans and non-binary youth

Is it any wonder that data demonstrates that when people respect the gender of trans and non-binary people, and when trans folks have access to connection, employment, education, housing, and healthcare, their health outcomes improve dramatically? For example, researchers from The Trevor Project found that "transgender and non-binary . . . youth who reported gender identity acceptance from at least one adult had 33% lower odds of reporting a past-year suicide attempt." Another study published in the *Journal of Adolescent Medicine* reported that "an increase by one context (i.e., home, school, work, or with friends) in which a chosen name could be used predicted a 5.37-unit decrease in depressive symptoms, a 29% decrease in suicidal ideation, and a 56% decrease in suicidal behavior."

Access to puberty-blocking medications or hormones that initiate the correct puberty has been shown to provide lifetime protection against suicide. And, according to the Family Acceptance Project, even in the face of extensive institutional discrimination, family acceptance has the most significant protective effect against homelessness, incarceration, tobacco smoking, drug and alcohol use, anxiety, depression, and suicidal behaviors. (You can read much more about the Family Acceptance Project at https://familyproject.sfsu.edu.)

Some therapeutic approaches that have been used successfully by patients and clinicians attempting to treat trauma and post-traumatic stress disorder (PTSD) include cognitive processing therapy, prolonged exposure therapy, dialectical behavior therapy, and internal family systems therapy. Some folks have found relief with different types of psychiatric medications, and PTSD is a qualifying condition for medical cannabis patients in many areas of the United States (https://www.mpp.org/issues/medical-marijuana/ptsd-medical-cannabis-programs/). Studies on psychedelic treatments for stress and trauma date back to the 1960s, and current research indicates that some psychedelic drugs, like psilocybin, MDMA, and ketamine, show real potential to be effective in this area.

Many successful treatments for trauma are accessed through a professional therapist (see Chapter 12 for more information on finding a therapist locally or online). The following trauma treatments are showing real promise:

>> **Art, music, play, and animal-assisted therapies:** All these therapeutic methods attempt to reach the part of the brain that's beyond the verbal processing of trauma.

>> **Cognitive behavioral therapy (CBT):** CBT is talk therapy provided by a licensed therapist that helps you recognize and process negative thoughts

and behavior (https://www.apa.org/ptsd-guideline/treatments/cognitive-behavioral-therapy).

>> **Emotional Freedom Techniques (EFT) tapping:** Anxiety can be reduced with EFT by tapping pressure points across your body (https://tinyurl.com/nyjyndsw).

>> **Eye movement desensitization and reprocessing (EMDR) therapy:** Provided by a licensed and trained therapist, EMDR therapy involves focusing on an external stimulus, such as moving your eyes in certain ways or paddles that buzz your hands, as you process traumatic memories and feelings (https://www.emdr.com/what-is-emdr/). It has a great track record for treating PTSD.

>> **Mindfulness:** This includes meditation and yoga. Don't be intimidated or fall for the mistaken belief that mindfulness is mystical nonsense! Meditation may not be exactly what you think it is, and even a few minutes a day can change your mind. Some apps and websites that can help you practice mindfulness are Smiling Mind (https://www.smilingmind.com.au/), Insight Timer (https://insighttimer.com/), and Psych Central (https://psychcentral.com/health/what-is-trauma-informed-yoga#trauma-informed-teaching).

>> **Somatic therapy:** This newer, but very promising, approach uses a mind-body connection to treat trauma (https://www.choosingtherapy.com/somatic-therapy/).

Addressing Simple Aesthetics and Hygiene Basics

Some of the following personal care and hygiene-related aspects of transition have been written about and discussed extensively, in person and online, by trans and non-binary people. Others are more overlooked or forgotten. If any of these healthcare-adjacent issues and treatments apply to you, they probably feel really important. Here's some info about aesthetics, or esthetics, and hygiene concerns.

Removing hair

You have quite a few options for removing body hair that you don't love. For use at home, you can purchase waxing kits, sugaring supplies, depilatory creams (like the old standby Nair), and even at-home laser hair removal devices.

The at-home lasers haven't been shown to be as effective as the ones utilized by trained, licensed professionals, but they may be worth a shot if you live a long way from a facility that provides this treatment.

Professional estheticians use wax, sugar, and even threading to remove hair from your face and body. Laser hair removal and electrolysis performed by licensed professionals can have longer-lasting results. Each method has some potential challenges, mainly temporary redness and blisters shortly after the treatment.

Both laser and electrolysis are notoriously painful. If you're concerned about the discomfort, you may want to experiment with topical anesthetics containing *lidocaine* (a numbing agent). You can read more about laser hair removal and electrolysis online at https://transcare.ucsf.edu/guidelines/hair-removal.

REMEMBER

If you're trans masculine or non-binary, you may also have strong feelings about removing unwanted hair from your face or your body. Hair removal is often discussed, and even marketed, as a service for women, both trans and cis. But anyone can dislike the hair growth patterns on their face or body and want to change them.

Handling common hygiene issues

Consistently following healthy hygiene practices can be challenging for some folks, for many different reasons. People who are *neurodivergent* (have brains that work differently than what is called "typical," for example, autistic or ADHD), especially those with ADHD, report difficulties with maintaining a regular toothbrushing habit. And people who are struggling with substance misuse, which is an issue for lots of trans and non-binary folks, have reported neglecting different aspects of their hygiene. When you factor in gender dysphoria, you can see how healthy hygiene habits may be a serious issue for some people.

If you haven't been able to keep up with your hygiene for any reason, it's not too late to start. Seeing a dentist, getting a haircut — especially one that's gender-affirming — washing your hair, and taking care of your skin can start today.

Brushing and flossing your teeth

Brushing and flossing your teeth isn't gendered behavior and doesn't involve gendered products for the most part. But some people have stated that being able to transition and represent themself as the gender they really are has given them new confidence and new energy to focus on their health, well-being, and appearance.

You can read a good article from the Mayo Clinic about the importance of oral hygiene to your overall health (https://tinyurl.com/5xnfcb27), and you may find it helpful — and even a bit surprising — to watch a short video from the American Dental Association about how to properly brush your teeth (https://tinyurl.com/3ar8mbtu).

Caring for your fingernails

Taking care of your fingernails is another aspect of personal hygiene that can change if you undergo hormone therapy or transition. Although no outcomes are universal, many folks who take estrogen report that their nails become more fragile and brittle over time. Moisturizing your nails and caring for your nail bed can help if you're experiencing dry, brittle fingernails and trying to grow your nails longer (https://tinyurl.com/bddf3ywj).

TIP

Any person of any gender can enjoy acrylic nails, nail art, manicures, and more. Fingernail polish itself has shed many of the gendered associations of the past, with even super masculine athletes painting their fingernails these days. So if you love having fingernails that are more stereotypically feminine, go for it!

Minimizing potentially offensive body odors

Taking hormones changes your body odors to a surprising degree. Not only is this true about your sweaty armpits, but it's also true about any other areas of your body that typically have a stronger scent, like your genitals and feet. Rest assured that it's normal and natural to have some body odor.

Although you may experience *gender euphoria* (happiness and excitement that your sex and gender match) from these changing smells, in modern culture, people share an expectation that body odors will be minimized in situations that bring them close together, especially in a work setting. Using a good soap and deodorant should be all you need to keep your natural scent at a socially acceptable level.

REMEMBER

For some people, finally being able to purchase and use highly gendered hygiene products is a treat, although others find these products part of the problem. Trans masculine and trans feminine people may not be attracted to the stereotypical scents associated with those genders. And many non-binary people say that their difficulties in culturally navigating gender are compounded by the seemingly inflexible nature of gendered products. Luckily, these days, alternatives are available.

The Good Trade highlights some current companies that make non-gendered hygiene products (https://www.thegoodtrade.com/features/gender-neutral-skincare/). Even relatively mainstream brands like Tom's of Maine and Schmidt's offer scents that can be perceived as unisex. And, in truth, if you love a soap or deodorant that's marketed at a gender different from your own, go ahead and use it. They don't check ID at the cash register to make sure a woman isn't buying Old Spice or a man isn't buying Secret.

TIP

Speak to your healthcare provider, or even your friends or support group, if soap and deodorant aren't doing the job on their own. Folks who have figured this issue out will have advice about products or approaches that work for them.

Facing a different skincare routine

Your face hygiene can also evolve as you move forward into both hormone treatment and aging. Many people experience at least some degree of acne during the first few years of hormone treatment, because you're essentially activating puberty when you change the balance of your hormonal system. We talk more about this in Chapter 8, but for now just know that taking testosterone increases both the oiliness of your skin and the possibility of acne. Over time, estrogen-based treatment softens the skin and doesn't create as much oil, but puberty is puberty, and in the first few years, folks using estrogen therapy may have to contend with some acne.

In general, the same acne treatments that are proven and successful for cisgender people, especially those aimed at adolescents, are a good bet for treating any acne you encounter during your first few years of hormone treatment. WebMD offers some basic tips for preventing acne at https://tinyurl.com/53avebn7.

Dealing with menstruation

We saved the most difficult hygiene topic for last: menstruation. Because every trans and non-binary person is different, we know that some people who were designated female at birth truly don't mind the monthly fact of getting a period, and some people may even enjoy it. However, a large number of trans masculine folks find menstruating incredibly dysphoric, with some reporting that they feel *dissociative* (mentally disconnected or detached) about it.

REMEMBER

Although there's an increased focus on using gender-neutral language about many things (for instance, check out this brief article from the hilariously named period product company Aunt Flow at https://tinyurl.com/ywmf3bs5), no alternate, gender-neutral word for menstruation itself has yet emerged.

Some trans and non-binary people seek out options that stop menstruation. Testosterone (or T) therapy, has that benefit for almost everyone who decides to take it. Surgery that removes the uterus and/or ovaries is a permanent solution that some choose. But many people, who either don't want to take T or aren't ready for hormone therapy or surgery just yet, opt for products that are typically sold as birth control medication. The most common of these options for delaying or stopping menstruation are

>> Birth control pill

>> Hormonal intrauterine device (or IUD for short)

>> DMPA contraceptive injection (such as Depo-Provera)

>> Vaginal ring (such as NuvaRing)

Each method has pros and cons, especially if you're coming at them from a place of gender dysphoria. The Mayo Clinic outlines the basics of hormonal birth control in an informative online article (https://tinyurl.com/3jbvkf2m), and you should absolutely be able to talk to your healthcare provider about your choices for stopping or delaying menstruation and the risks and benefits for you. Another great resource is your closest Planned Parenthood clinic.

TIP

Some companies make all kinds of period products that are meant to be gender-neutral or gender-affirming. TomboyX (https://tomboyx.com/collections/period-underwear) offers underwear especially for periods, including shorts and what they call "boy shorts" that aren't actually gendered. And an article at The Cut provides an overview of additional gender-neutral period products (https://www.thecut.com/article/best-period-products-trans-nonbinary.html).

IN THIS CHAPTER

» **Preparing for hormone treatment**

» **Taking masculinizing hormones and what to expect**

» **Taking feminizing hormones and what to expect**

» **Engaging with hormones in a genderfluid way**

» **Examining gender-affirming medical care for kids**

Chapter **8**

Opting for Hormone Therapy

When we talk about hormone therapy or hormone treatment, we're referring to the process of using what are called *exogenous* (a big word that just means external, or coming from the outside) hormones to change your *hormonal milieu* (the combination of hormones in your body). Some transgender men and *trans masculine people* (an umbrella term that covers transgender men and anyone who has a masculine gender that differs from their designated sex) choose to bring testosterone into their bodies from the outside, because the body they were born with doesn't make testosterone as the predominant sex hormone. Likewise, some transgender women and trans feminine people choose to bring estrogen into their bodies from the outside (and block the testosterone), because the body they were born with doesn't make estrogen as the predominant sex hormone.

TIP

Gender is a spectrum, and your goals for hormone therapy are part of your personal gender journey. Trans men, trans women, and non-binary people can have different and/or overlapping desires about the potential outcomes of hormone therapy. Talk to your healthcare provider about what's possible.

In this chapter, you get a great deal of information about how hormones work. You also find out about all the different methods for taking hormones, as well as the typical changes you can expect from them. Some of those changes may sound great, while others may sound like things you don't really want. You can talk to your healthcare provider about how to most effectively get the results you're looking for. Sometimes you can't achieve one outcome without others, but sometimes you can. You may be anxious to make the changes you're expecting, so we also cover the timeline of typical changes from hormone treatment.

Because non-binary people sometimes want and need hormones, too, we talk a bit about low-dose hormone therapy Finally, you find some details about hormone treatment and puberty-blocking medications for young people.

Knowing What Happens Before You Start Hormone Therapy

Hormone treatment or hormone therapy can be a *huge* step for trans and non-binary people, if it's the right fit. It's sometimes pursued for health reasons (for instance testosterone can be part of a treatment regimen for Ehlers-Danlos Syndrome — a connective tissue disorder), but often it's one of the key options that helps some people finally feel like the person they always knew they were meant to be.

That feeling of congruence, confidence, or becoming your real self, comes from the development of desired (and suppression of unwanted) *secondary sex characteristics*, traits that are typically derived from a person's biological sex and aren't involved in reproductive function, such as pubic and facial hair growth and breast development. In this case, the traits don't come from biological sex but from the use of hormone therapy.

Sometimes, even before people see any external changes, they feel really amazing internal changes that they describe as more aligned with their gender. How hormone treatment works for you depends on your genetics and the dosing of your hormones, but when you take hormones at the most common therapeutic dose, you induce puberty. That may not sound like fun (and sometimes it really isn't) but just like a teenager, you have to go through this developmental period to reach your personal goals. This may sound intimidating, but in the end, a lot of trans folks talk about finally loving to look in the mirror once the hormones start to work their magic.

Your goals for taking hormones will be as individual as you are. For some people, the idea is to take a dose that will initiate the puberty that's right for them, and obtain all the secondary sex characteristics possible. Other people are hoping for some of these traits but not others. For instance, you can take testosterone at a low dose, which can improve your mood and energy and even help with muscle growth and development, but need to stop short of more typically masculine hair growth — on the face and body.

Before we get into more detail about masculinizing and feminizing hormone treatments, you should know what to expect before you begin hormone therapy. At the start, your healthcare provider will likely perform a comprehensive evaluation process. This often includes

>> **Going over mental health criteria for gender dysphoria:** Your provider will ensure that you meet clinical guidelines for *gender dysphoria* (feelings of discomfort because your body doesn't match your internal sense of your gender).

>> **Getting informed consent:** You and your provider will discuss which hormone therapy involves, along with its potential risks and side effects.

>> **Evaluating your mental health:** Your provider will assess whether any untreated psychiatric issues affect your ability to make safe, informed medical decisions. This is rare but can be a reason for delaying treatment.

>> **Doing baseline blood work:** Your provider will order blood work to check for any physical issues that can complicate hormone therapy, including abnormal liver function, cholesterol levels, and hormone levels like testosterone and estradiol.

>> **Screening for hormone-sensitive cancers:** Some cancers, such as breast or ovarian cancer, are sensitive to hormonal changes and need to be ruled out before you can start hormones. (You can find more info on this at https://www.webmd.com/breast-cancer/hormone-sensitive-cancers.)

REMEMBER

Transgender and non-binary people, just like *cisgender* people (whose gender identity matches their sex assigned at birth), can have psychiatric and behavioral health issues that shouldn't interfere with their ability to make decisions about their treatment. A healthcare provider should only be wary of moving forward with hormone therapy if they believe that your issues prevent you from making an informed, independent decision, which is pretty darn rare.

Starting Masculinizing Hormones

Masculinizing hormone therapy has one component: testosterone. Exogenous testosterone, or T, as it's often called, is a powerful estrogen suppressor, and for most patients it causes menstrual periods to stop, so there's no clinical need to suppress estrogen, even if you still have ovaries or a uterus. The biggest variable in testosterone therapy is the dosing, which is usually based on the changes you're hoping to achieve from taking it.

Many folks wish that there was some available treatment that would allow their body to produce its own testosterone, in other words to have functional testes. For transgender men, this is not possible at this time. You can currently opt for testicular implants, which are made of silicone and meant to give the appearance of the type of scrotum and testicles a cisgender man may have. So far, nobody has figured out any treatments that can give a transgender or non-binary person the reproductive organs or capabilities that many — but not all — cisgender folks have.

REMEMBER

If you were designated female at birth, no currently available treatment will enable your body to produce sperm or semen or contribute to a pregnancy from that side of the reproductive process. Who knows what the future holds? But today, if you were designated female at birth and you want or need any of the effects of testosterone, you have to use exogenous T.

WARNING

There's still mixed evidence about the long-term health or safety concerns of taking hormones as part of gender-affirming care. However, most knowledgeable healthcare providers view hormone therapy as a way of starting the body's "true puberty" and maintaining the right hormonal balance for someone's accurate gender.

Anticipating changes and timelines

What are the changes that testosterone can create in the body? You'll see quite a few, including

>> **Changes to skin (begins from 1–6 months):** Taking testosterone can increase your skin's oil production, causing acne. See Chapter 7 for more info and tips on managing this issue.

>> **Increased body/facial hair growth (begins from 3–6 months):** How much new hair you'll grow depends on your genetics. Your beard and body hair patterns are determined by your family of origin and your genes. Some guys have thick, full beards, while others have only a few whiskers. If you check them out, you'll see this is true for cis guys, too.

>> **Male-pattern baldness (begins from 6–12 months):** Baldness is also completely genetic. Some treatments and medications, such as finasteride (interestingly also used in a different dose by trans feminine people to block testosterone more broadly), are very successful at stopping hair loss, so don't be afraid to ask for help at the first signs of a receding hairline, if it bothers you.

>> **Increased libido (begins from 1–6 months):** While a higher sex drive may sound fun, it can be quite intense in those first couple of years of puberty. Going through puberty again varies from person to person, so try not to overthink some of these changes.

>> **Clitoral growth (begins from 3–6 months):** Testosterone's effect on the clitoris can be pretty remarkable, and it's considered one of the irreversible effects of taking testosterone. The healthcare website FOLX has some great information, illustrations, and even an animation (go to https://www.folxhealth.com/library/testosterone-bottom-growth).

>> **Vaginal atrophy (begins from 1–6 months):** This term sounds, admittedly, a little dramatic. *Vaginal atrophy* is more accurately described as vaginal dryness, which causes the tissue of the vagina to become thinner and more fragile with testosterone use. It can also result in decreased lubrication. Simple treatments like topical estrogen cream applied directly to the vaginal walls can help if you experience this sometimes painful issue or if it causes any challenges in your sex life.

>> **Fat loss/redistribution (begins from 1–6 months):** You won't automatically lose weight when you start testosterone, but many people report a higher metabolism and more ease in losing weight. It's also common for people to see fat deposits on the body move around to more stereotypical areas for their gender. For example, people taking T often see fat move from the thighs and hips to the belly area.

Remember that these are generalizations. Just like cis men's, trans folks' bodies are incredibly different from one person to the next.

WARNING

>> **Increased muscle mass/strength (begins from 6–12 months):** Many people say that after they take testosterone, they notice they have more upper-body strength, even if they don't work out or exercise. For people who do work out, the difference when on testosterone is usually profound. You'll probably notice intensified returns on your exercise investment!

>> **Period/menstruation interruption (begins from 1–6 months):** Some people experience breakthrough bleeding on T, but for a lot of people, testosterone therapy on its own is enough to stop their body from having a period. This effect depends on the level of testosterone in your blood, so if your bleeding returns, tell your healthcare provider so that you can get labs to check what's happening. Remember that even if your periods stop,

testosterone is *never* protection against pregnancy (or duh! against sexually transmitted infections).

>> **Changes in emotions and social engagement (begins from 1-6 months):** This is definitely not a foregone conclusion, but some people talk about having a harder time crying, especially in the early years of taking hormones/experiencing puberty. Others report differences in the way they relate to people. While this is a possible outcome, you don't want to be too swayed by gender stereotypes when you anticipate the changes you'll experience.

>> **Deeper voice (begins from 6–12 months):** This varies from person to person and probably has a genetic component as well. Just like trans women and trans feminine people, trans men and trans masculine folks can have voice training/speech therapy to develop a deeper tone of voice if desired.

REMEMBER

For most people, these changes begin within the timeline outlined in parentheses in the preceding list. But many effects of testosterone take years to reach their peak. For example, from start to finish, growing a full beard can often take 3–4 years, just like for a cis boy going through puberty.

Figure 8-1 shows a table that lists all of these changes, along with the timelines. It also indicates which traits are reversible and which are not.

EFFECTS AND EXPECTED TIME COURSE OF TESTOSTERONE

The degree and rate of physical effects is dependent on the dose and route of administration, as well as patient-specific factors such as age, genetics, body habitus and lifestyle. Hormone therapy results in both reversible and irreversible masculinization.

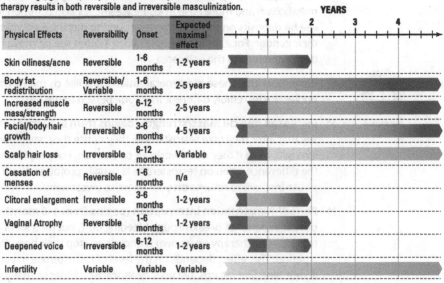

Physical Effects	Reversibility	Onset	Expected maximal effect
Skin oiliness/acne	Reversible	1-6 months	1-2 years
Body fat redistribution	Reversible/Variable	1-6 months	2-5 years
Increased muscle mass/strength	Reversible	6-12 months	2-5 years
Facial/body hair growth	Irreversible	3-6 months	4-5 years
Scalp hair loss	Irreversible	6-12 months	Variable
Cessation of menses	Reversible	1-6 months	n/a
Clitoral enlargement	Irreversible	3-6 months	1-2 years
Vaginal Atrophy	Reversible	1-6 months	1-2 years
Deepened voice	Irreversible	6-12 months	1-2 years
Infertility	Variable	Variable	Variable

FIGURE 8-1: Some changes and timelines associated with masculinizing hormones. (Credit: https://www.rainbowhealthontario.ca)

Choosing a delivery method

Can you get your hormones from Instacart? No! But that would be cool. What we mean by *delivery method* is the way you get exogenous hormones into your body and bloodstream. You can choose between several methods of taking testosterone, including the following:

>> **Intramuscular injection:** With this method, you inject the testosterone into your muscle tissue (usually the thigh or the butt muscle).

>> **Subcutaneous injection:** This involves injecting T into the layer of fat right under the skin (usually in the belly). And this is just as effective as intramuscular and requires a smaller injection needle.

>> **Transdermal patches:** These self-adhesive patches that deliver T through contact with the skin are manufactured by pharmaceutical companies. These are made more for cis men with low testosterone levels and don't seem to work as well as the injections and topical gels.

>> **Transdermal gel:** The pharmaceutical companies make testosterone gel under brand names like AndroGel. You apply the gel to your skin according to your healthcare provider's instructions.

>> **Compounded testosterone gel:** You may have a local compounding pharmacy that can prepare your testosterone gel on-site, to your provider's specifications. Compounded medicines are often not covered by insurance, but they have some benefits compared to standard pharmaceuticals (such as a higher concentration in a lower volume of medication) and can be more affordable than using insurance. In some places, compounded testosterone is about $120 for a 6-month supply.

Why would you choose one method over another? There's a lot of debate in the trans masculine community about which method is the "best," but the most important thing is which one is best for you. Some people really hate the idea of giving themselves injections of any kind, while others are comfortable doing the small-needle subcutaneous (also called *Sub-Q* or *SQ*) injections, but not the intramuscular injections using much larger needles. Still others may find the daily routine of using gel hard to remember, and much prefer the often weekly dosing via injection. Your dosing method may also be tied to your personal desires for the hormone therapy. Many non-binary people microdose which *can* be easier with gel or topical application.

Some people have reported that their bodies had difficulty absorbing and metabolizing the gel and they have to inject testosterone to get their levels high enough in their lab tests (see the next section for dosing info). As you'd probably guess, there can be some trial and error in the process. You and your provider will work it out.

Even if you find the perfect delivery method and dose for you, things may change over time because of factors like aging and illness, for example.

Determining your dose

How much testosterone you should start with or take regularly is a very common question. The answer depends on your goals for hormone therapy. We cover what can be called non-binary or more genderfluid goals later in this chapter (see "Achieving Gender-Expansive Hormone Goals"). In this section, we discuss what has been considered for many years the typical masculinizing course of testosterone therapy, in which you go through male puberty and emerge with whatever masculine secondary sex characteristics your genetics support.

Your testosterone dose is determined by the results of your blood tests, but typical recommendations for starting doses of injectable testosterone (testosterone enanthate or testosterone cypionate, depending on the carrier oil the T is floating in) are 30–50 milligrams (mg) per week. There's really no maximum dosage as long as you and your healthcare provider are tracking the testosterone level in your blood.

Adjustments to your dosage will occur near the beginning of your hormone therapy. Your provider will probably increase or decrease your dose by 10 mg at a time if you need to go up or down. Any dose can be split in half to more evenly spread out the effects of the testosterone if you tolerate that better. Some people have said that they start to feel bad — for instance, experiencing headaches, mood swings, or even breakthrough period bleeding — if their injections are spaced too far apart. Much more info about each type of delivery method and dose is available at https://transcare.ucsf.edu/guidelines/masculinizing-therapy.

It's important to take into account both your experience with how the hormones are working and your lab results that show the testosterone levels in your bloodstream when making decisions with your healthcare provider about how to *titrate* (move up or down) your dose of hormones. The clinical guidelines indicate that the range for maximized masculinization is between 400 and 1,000 nanograms (ng) of testosterone per deciliter (dL) of blood. Both your experience and your lab results are important because if your provider only checks how you're feeling without doing blood work, your serum level may be lower than the typical range, holding you back from your goals.

When your serum testosterone is below 400 ng/dL for too long, your bone health may suffer, and if your level is way above 1,000 ng/dL, your body may convert the testosterone into estradiol. Way back in 2006, a small study of 31 transgender men newly started on either 50–60 mg/week subcutaneous testosterone cypionate, 5 grams/day 1% testosterone gel or 4 mg/day testosterone patch found that after

6 months, 21 of the subjects (68 percent) achieved male-range testosterone levels and 5 (16 percent) had persistent menstrual periods, with only 9 (29 percent) having normal male-range estradiol levels.

In other words, even if you're on a typical dose of T, your body may not be getting to the right testosterone level. That's why the dose is less important to focus on than your blood level. The first year, your healthcare provider may check your T level as often as every 3 months, but once you get to the right level, annual labs should be sufficient.

WARNING

Taking the maximum dose doesn't guarantee getting the maximum masculinizing effects. And it's critical to understand that taking more testosterone than your body needs can cause a range of negative side effects, from mood swings to increased period bleeding. This is because a percentage of testosterone is always converted to estrogen in your body, so if you're taking excess T, that percentage will be higher. Maximum masculinizing effects come from your T level being in the 400–1,000 ng/dL range over time and your body being able to produce masculine secondary sex characteristics in response to the T.

Being aware of possible risks

Several potential risks or side effects have been anecdotally linked to testosterone use (meaning they've been individually reported by users), but the research so far hasn't nailed down any connections. So, the following list of *possible* risks hasn't been verified at this point. However, some concerns that warrant further study to confirm or deny include

>> Higher cholesterol

>> Stroke and cardiovascular disease

>> Increased risk of diabetes

>> Weight gain

>> Onset or worsening of migraines

>> Changes to autoimmune conditions

Again, no long-term studies have provided clear answers about any of these possible side effects. We include them here for your information.

One risk that's pretty well documented at this point is a thickening of the blood, also called *erythrocytosis* or *polycythemia*. This can cause a high *hematocrit* (red blood cell) count, which may result in strokes, heart attacks, and other cardiovascular consequences. Donating blood occasionally seems to control this side effect, and being on the correct dose of testosterone also helps. And to be clear, just being on T doesn't lead to heart attacks.

TIP

If your red blood cell counts are high over time, you can get an evaluation for *sleep apnea* (a condition that causes you to stop breathing when you sleep), and you should cut back or quit if you use tobacco products. Anything that makes your body think it's not getting enough oxygen will make your red blood cell level go up.

Another clear side effect of taking testosterone is acne. Breakouts can peak in the first year for some people, but for others severe acne may continue for years. Because everyone's experience is different, the tendency to develop acne while you're taking T seems to be at least in part genetic. Most of the time, you can get relief with over-the-counter treatments. If that doesn't work for you, talk to your healthcare provider about prescription solutions.

Using Feminizing Hormones

Trans feminine folks currently don't have any way to obtain the type of *gonads* (internal reproductive organs) that would create the right hormone balance for them. If you were designated male at birth, no treatment available today will enable your body to make its own estrogen, become pregnant, or carry a baby. (But again, who knows what the future holds.) If you were designated male at birth and you want or need any of the effects of estrogen, you have to use exogenous estrogen. If you still have your testes, you also have to take an antiandrogen to medically block the testosterone in your body and allow the estrogen to work for you.

Feminizing hormone therapy has at least two components: taking estrogen and blocking testosterone. Some folks also report beneficial results from using progesterone, which we discuss in the following section.

Anticipating changes and timelines

Estrogen can create quite a few changes in your body, including the following:

>> **Changes to skin (begins from 3–6 months):** Taking estrogen decreases oil production in your sebaceous glands, resulting in softer skin. Many see this change first and *love* it! While acne isn't a typical side effect of feminizing therapy, you may see increased acne during the first few years, just because of the whole return-to-puberty thing. See Chapter 7 for more info and tips on managing this hygiene issue.

» **Decreased body/facial hair growth (begins from 6–12 months):** Feminizing therapy won't cause your facial or body hair to just fall out, but it will thin it and slow its growth. Only permanent hair removal gets rid of body and facial hair for good. Check out Chapter 7 for more in-depth information about hair removal.

» **End to scalp hair loss (begins from 1–3 months):** Unfortunately, taking estrogen cannot help you grow new hair, but any pattern baldness you're experiencing should stop.

» **Breast growth (begins from 3–6 months):** For many people, growing breasts is one of the most exciting effects of estrogen therapy. Initial breast growth, sometimes called *breast buds,* can be tender or even a little painful. Growth varies from person to person — most likely because of genetics — so expect your outcome to be different from other people's.

» **Decreased sperm production (variable):** Feminizing therapy causes sperm production to decline significantly or even completely stop. The research isn't clear about whether going off hormone therapy for 3–6 months can cause sperm production to bounce back, so some experts recommend making decisions about hormone therapy based on the assumption that it won't. Chapter 11 covers more details about family planning, including the preservation of sperm.

» **Decreased testicular volume (begins from 3–6 months):** Because sperm production is reduced, the size of your testicles can shrink by as much as half. If you're planning on genital surgery, the amount of scrotal skin you have won't change, and it will be available for future surgical procedures.

» **Less frequent spontaneous erections (begins from 1–3 months):** Feminizing therapy contributes to a decrease in spontaneous erections. If you do have an erection, it may not be hard enough to penetrate someone else sexually. This is another effect of hormone therapy that feels like a major relief to some folks. If you don't feel that way, medications that treat erectile dysfunction (for example, sildenafil/Viagra) can work for you, too. While you may think of these drugs as being only for men, women and non-binary folks have used them to great success too.

» **Decreased libido (begins from 1–3 months):** Some people say they have a lower sex drive during feminizing hormone therapy. This can be something you celebrate, or it may be an unwanted side effect.

» **Body fat redistribution (begins from 3–6 months):** It's common for people to see fat deposits on the body move around to more stereotypical areas for their gender. For example, people taking estrogen often see fat move from the midsection to the hips and thighs.

Remember, these side effects are generalizations. Just like with cis women's, trans women's bodies are incredibly different from one person to the next.

>> **Decreased muscle mass/strength (begins from 3–6 months):** Estrogen causes an overall decrease in muscle mass, and trans feminine people on hormone therapy sometimes report not being able to do things they previously did in terms of lifting heavy objects or doing pull-ups (which may not have been your thing before). Again, you don't want to get too caught up in gender stereotypes — remember, cis and trans women compete at the elite levels of most sports these days! But overall, people do talk about decreased strength as an effect of feminizing hormones.

>> **Changes in emotions and social engagement (begins from 1-6 months):** This is definitely not a foregone conclusion, but some people talk about experiencing different feelings or relating to others in different ways once the hormonal makeup of their body shifts. Emotional and social changes can be especially noticeable in the early years of taking hormones/experiencing puberty. While this is a possible outcome, you don't want to get too tapped into gender stereotypes when you anticipate the changes you'll experience. One person described starting feminizing hormones like this: "I've been looking at a pamphlet of a museum my whole life, and now I'm seeing it in person. So of course I'm more emotional! And it feels so affirming."

The proverbial jury is still out, but some trans feminine people say that taking the hormone progesterone helps with stabilizing mood swings as well as developing rounder, though not larger, breasts. Reliable studies don't exist to back this up, but if you want to try it, your healthcare provider may start you on 100 mg of daily bioidentical (identical on a molecular level with endogenous hormones) progesterone (Prometrium). Your provider may tell you that it can decrease your estradiol serum levels, which just means you need to make sure to get regular checkups. There are no labs to check progesterone levels, and if no changes are obvious even with a 200 mg dose, it's probably not worth taking progesterone.

Unfortunately, you can't change your voice through hormone use. If testosterone lowered your voice during *natal puberty* (puberty during your teens), that's one of the more permanent changes. A surgical approach to raising voice pitch (discussed in more detail in Chapter 10) has received mixed reviews from patients. The more common and effective (and much less risky) option is voice training or vocal coaching, which is also covered in Chapter 10.

For most people, the changes brought on by estrogen therapy begin within the timeline outlined in parentheses in the list at the beginning of this section. Many effects of feminizing hormones take years to reach their peak. From start to finish, complete breast growth, or developing your personal curves, can often take 3–4 years, just like for cis girl going through puberty.

See Figure 8-2 for a table listing the changes you can expect from estrogen therapy, along with timelines. It also indicates which traits are reversible and which aren't.

EFFECTS AND EXPECTED TIME COURSE OF FEMINIZING HORMONES

The degree and rate of physical effects are largely dependent on patient-specific factors such as age, genetics, body habitus and lifestyle, and to some extent the dose and route used (selected in accordance with a patient's specific goals and risk profile).

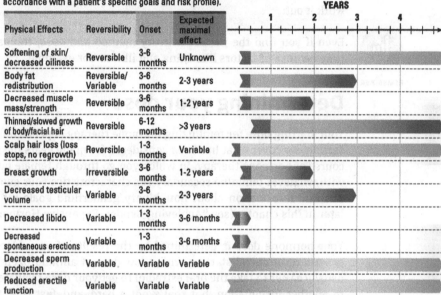

Physical Effects	Reversibility	Onset	Expected maximal effect
Softening of skin/decreased oiliness	Reversible	3-6 months	Unknown
Body fat redistribution	Reversible/Variable	3-6 months	2-3 years
Decreased muscle mass/strength	Reversible	3-6 months	1-2 years
Thinned/slowed growth of body/facial hair	Reversible	6-12 months	>3 years
Scalp hair loss (loss stops, no regrowth)	Reversible	1-3 months	Variable
Breast growth	Irreversible	3-6 months	1-2 years
Decreased testicular volume	Variable	3-6 months	2-3 years
Decreased libido	Variable	1-3 months	3-6 months
Decreased spontaneous erections	Variable	1-3 months	3-6 months
Decreased sperm production	Variable	Variable	Variable
Reduced erectile function	Variable	Variable	Variable

FIGURE 8-2: A table of the changes and timelines associated with feminizing hormones. (Credit: https://www.rainbow health ontario.ca)

Choosing a delivery method

So, how do you get exogenous hormones into your body and bloodstream? You can choose from the following delivery methods for your feminizing hormone therapy:

>> **Intramuscular injection:** This method requires weekly injections of estrogen into your muscle tissue (usually the thigh or the butt muscle).

>> **Subcutaneous injection:** This is a weekly injection into the layer of fat right under your skin (usually in the belly).

>> **Transdermal patches:** These self-adhesive patches manufactured by pharmaceutical companies deliver your estrogen dose through your skin.

>> **Oral pills:** Taking daily tablets is the most convenient delivery method for some people. This also means you get a highly regulated dose of antiandrogen and estrogen every day.

As with masculinizing hormone treatment, there's a lot of debate in the trans feminine community about which estrogen delivery method is the "best," but the most important thing is which one is best for you. Some people really hate the idea of giving themselves injections of any kind, while others are comfortable doing the small-needle subcutaneous injections, but not the intramuscular injections using much larger needles. Some folks may prefer a weekly injection because the patches don't stick well or cause a skin reaction or rash. As you'd probably expect, there can be some trial and error in the process. You and your provider will work it out.

Even if you find the perfect delivery method and dose, things can change over time because of factors like aging and illness, for example.

Determining your dose

Your starting dose for feminizing hormone therapy depends on your goals. In this section, we cover what has been considered for many years the typical feminizing course of hormone therapy, in which you go through female puberty and emerge with whatever feminine secondary sex characteristics your genetics support. You can find information about non-binary/genderfluid goals for hormone therapy later in this chapter (see "Achieving Gender-Expansive Hormone Goals").

Your hormone dose is determined by the results of your blood tests, but some experts recommend starting with a low dose of antiandrogen and estradiol. It's usually easier to take the oral estradiol to get your dose regulated and then switch to another formulation, but that's not a hard-and-fast rule. Some people start with 2 mg/day oral estradiol, or 3 mg/week injectable estradiol valerate, or 1–2 mg/week injectable estradiol cypionate, or a 0.05 mg/day transdermal patch once or twice a week. There's really no maximum dose of estrogen — the important thing is the level of estradiol and testosterone in your blood.

Antiandrogen therapy is most often administered through an oral medication called *spironolactone* or medications called *5-alpha reductase inhibitors,* which include finasteride and dutasteride tablets. The typical starting dose of spironolactone is 50 mg twice daily, and the maximum is 200 mg twice per day. For finasteride the starting dose is 1 mg per day, with a max of 5 mg daily. You can read more about these and other testosterone-blocking medical strategies online at https://transcare.ucsf.edu/guidelines/feminizing-hormone-therapy.

When making decisions with your healthcare provider about how to titrate your dose of hormones, it's important to take into account both your experience with how the hormones are working and your lab results that show the estradiol and testosterone levels in your bloodstream. According to the clinical guidelines, the range of serum estradiol levels for maximized femininization is between 100 and

200 picograms (pg) of estradiol per milliliter (mL) of blood, and the goal for serum testosterone, if full suppression is desired, is below 50 ng of testosterone per dL of blood. Both your experience and your lab results are important because if your provider only checks how you're feeling without doing blood work, your serum levels may be lower than the typical range, holding you back from your goals.

If your serum estradiol levels are below 100 pg/mL for 6 months to a year, your progress toward femininization will slow, and your bone health may decline. If your levels are way above 200 pg/mL, you may have a higher risk of getting blood clots in your legs and/or lungs. Data collected in 2015 showed that transgender women taking 4 mg/day divided dose oral estradiol or 100 micrograms transdermal estradiol, plus 100–200mg/day divided dose spironolactone, achieved normal female-range estradiol levels, though only two-thirds of them had female-range testosterone levels.

TOO MUCH OF A GOOD THING: HIGH DOSES OF HORMONES ARE RISKY

A common misconception is that higher doses of hormones will speed up physical changes during transition. But taking the maximum dose doesn't guarantee you'll get the maximum feminizing effects you want. And it's critical to understand that taking more estrogen than your body needs can cause a range of negative side effects.

Maddie Deutsch, a medical expert from the University of California, San Francisco (UCSF), cautions against this approach. She explains:

> Contrary to what many may have heard, you can achieve the maximum effect of your transition with doses of estrogen that result in your blood levels being similar to those of a pre-menopausal cisgender woman. Taking high doses does not necessarily make changes happen quicker. It could, however, endanger your health.

Deutsch also warns against overly complicated or intensive hormone regimens that promise dramatic results. These approaches aren't supported by current medical evidence, and higher estrogen levels beyond what's recommended don't enhance the feminizing effects of hormone therapy. Instead, the lack of testosterone is a more significant factor in achieving the desired results.

For more information, check out the UCSF Transgender Care Guidelines (https://transcare.ucsf.edu/article/information-estrogen-hormone-therapy).

In other words, one size doesn't fit all. A standardized dose of hormones isn't going to achieve the same outcome for you that someone else may see. The first year, your healthcare provider may check your hormone levels as often as every 3 months, but once you get to the right levels, annual labs should be sufficient.

Understanding the possible risks

Several potential risks or side effects have been anecdotally linked to estrogen use, but the research so far hasn't nailed down any connections. So, the following list of *possible* risks hasn't been verified at this point. However, some concerns that warrant further study to confirm or deny include

>> Risks of some cancers such as prostate and breast

>> Blood clots in your legs and/or lungs

>> Stroke and cardiovascular disease

>> Weight gain

>> Onset or worsening of migraines

>> Changes to autoimmune conditions

Again, no quality long-term studies have provided clear answers about any of these potential side effects. We include them here for your information.

One side effect of estrogen therapy that's pretty well documented is an elevated risk of blood clots (which is true for all people with higher levels of estradiol, including cis women compared to cis men), along with a risk of strokes and heart attacks, if you smoke cigarettes. Your healthcare provider will probably want to work with you on cutting back or quitting smoking to reduce your risk. Another way to lower your risk is to take your estrogen through the skin via a patch or gel.

It's also well-documented that hormone therapy affects fertility. Taking estrogen and antiandrogen dramatically decreases or fully halts sperm production and decreases testicle volume. While some people have regained the ability to produce sperm after stopping hormone treatment, that hasn't been the case for many others. Being on feminizing hormones doesn't protect against pregnancy. Check out Chapter 11 for more information on family planning.

TIP

If you have an *orchiectomy* (surgical removal of the testes) or a *vaginoplasty* (the surgical creation of a vagina, which involves removing the testes), you won't need to take the antiandrogen portion of your hormone therapy anymore. This medication suppresses the testosterone that your gonads make, so removing the gonads means you don't need it.

Achieving Gender-Expansive Hormone Goals

Some people who take estrogen or testosterone aren't trying to achieve maximized masculinization or feminization. For example, non-binary people may want or need the courses of hormone therapy described earlier in this chapter in order to develop all the secondary sex characteristics. And binary transgender people may be on a gender journey that doesn't involve gender dysphoria or medical treatment. Because each person truly is on their own gender journey or path (and that goes for cisgender folks too!), everyone's needs and goals are going to be a little bit different. Having said that, it isn't uncommon for non-binary people to use hormone therapy in a more genderfluid or gender-expansive way.

Gender-expansive goals can be achieved by using lower doses of hormone therapy, which some people call *microdosing*. You can follow the guidelines we outline for taking the different types of hormones (see the earlier section "Determining your dose") without aiming for the serum levels to reach maximized masculinization or femininization.

For non-binary masculinization the ideal serum testosterone level is as close to 400 ng/dL as possible. You'll probably find this easier to achieve with either low doses of daily topical testosterone or low doses of injectable testosterone administered twice a week to avoid dramatic swings in your hormone levels. If people on feminizing hormones are interested in non-binary outcomes and/or maintenance of sexual function, the serum estradiol goal is still between 100 and 200 pg/mL, and you can use an antiandrogen to achieve the desired testosterone level. If you decide to take lower doses of spironolactone to hang on to more sexual function, you may see fewer feminizing effects. You'll have to work with your healthcare provider to find the best balance.

WARNING

Once you're past 55, bone health becomes more of a concern for all people, but we don't have great data about "appropriate" serum levels at that age. While you and your provider should talk about bone health at that time, it will be up to you to determine what serum levels work for you since we don't have data for folks in the older (and wiser) age range. Even cisgender folks have to consider bone health more closely at this age and work with their medical providers to monitor and maintain healthy bones.

REMEMBER

Cisgender folks also use hormones for lots of reasons. Some cis women use estrogen and/or testosterone to mitigate some of the negative symptoms of menopause. Cis men use it for its anti-aging effects, or even at a younger age for increased energy and libido. There are also some cis folks who use these hormones to masculinize or feminize in a gender expansive way, too. They do not identify as trans but do want some of these physical changes as gender goals.

Providing Treatment for Trans and Non-Binary Children

A common misconception these days is that young children have access to (and a need for) all different kinds of transition-related medical treatments, including hormone therapy. Of course this isn't true, but what *are* the medical options for trans and non-binary kids?

SUPPORTING YOUNG TRANS AND NON-BINARY CHILDREN WITHOUT SURGERY OR HORMONES

Children as young as 5 can have a clear sense of their gender, according to the American Academy of Pediatrics. But does that mean a young trans or non-binary child needs surgery or medical intervention? No! For young trans and non-binary children, the focus should be on social and emotional support, not medical or surgical procedures.

Key elements of social and emotional support include allowing children to explore their identity by

- Choosing their clothing
- Picking their hairstyle
- Selecting their name and pronouns

This process, known as *social transition*, has been shown to positively impact mental health outcomes. A 2021 study from Fenway Health found that people who socially transitioned early in their childhood were less likely to use substances like marijuana later in life, suggesting that they had lower anxiety levels compared to those who waited until adulthood to socially transition.

In addition, working with a gender-affirming medical provider early on is essential. These providers can offer support by using the right name and pronouns, being sensitive to the child's view of their body, and making accommodations during medical exams to ensure a comfortable experience.

For more information, see the Fenway Health study (https://www.sciencedirect.com/science/article/abs/pii/S1054139X21002834?dgcid=coauthor).

When natal puberty begins, a lot of trans and non-binary youths experience extreme levels of distress. While puberty can be a tough time for many young people, the physical changes it brings can send trans and non-binary kids into a real psychological tailspin. Luckily, trans youths have a safe way to press the pause button on puberty.

Considering puberty blockers

Puberty blockers suspend pubertal development, which can decrease gender dysphoria and give kids and their families time to navigate their gender and their gender journey. Typically, trans and non-binary kids are considered eligible for these treatments if they have consistently demonstrated that they feel like a different gender, are able to make their own decisions, and have been informed of the medication's effects and side effects and given information and options about fertility.

Medically, puberty blockers are known as *GnRH agonists*, and they're delivered through monthly injections or a small *subdermal implant* (a very small pellet of medication placed under the skin that releases slowly over 6–12 months). The treatment needs to be started by Tanner stage 2 or Tanner stage 3, which typically occur between the ages of 8 and 13. (The *Tanner stages* mark the progression of puberty in the body. You can find more information about the various stages of puberty at `https://www.healthline.com/health/parenting/stages-of-puberty`.)

A child receiving puberty blockers can't have any medical conditions that would cause issues with the treatment, and they're encouraged, but not required, to receive behavioral health support. You can find clinical information about the dosing and monitoring of GnRH agonists in the Endocrine Society's 2017 guidelines on the treatment of gender dysphoria (`https://www.endocrine.org/clinical-practice-guidelines/gender-dysphoria-gender-incongruence`).

Based on all the medical evidence involving trans kids, puberty suppression appears to be completely reversible. However, the long-term effects of puberty blockers on bone health and fertility are not completely known, so those factors should be considered in the decision-making process.

Puberty suppressors have been shown to have a positive impact on the life outcomes of the people who've used them (`https://growinguptransgender.com/2020/06/10/puberty-blockers-overview-of-the-research/`). One commonly cited Dutch study found that "a whopping 98% of people who had started gender-affirming medical treatment in adolescence continued to use gender-affirming hormones at follow-up"(`https://www.npr.org/2022/10/26/1131398960/gender-affirming-care-trans-puberty-suppression-teens`).

Lastly, an important American study demonstrated lifetime protection against suicidality provided by access to pubertal suppression (https://pmc.ncbi.nlm.nih.gov/articles/PMC7073269/).

The benefits of this therapy may include

» Improving mental health and well-being

» Reducing depression and anxiety

» Improving social interaction with peers

» Eliminating need for future gender-affirming procedures

» Reducing thoughts or actions related to self-harm

REMEMBER

In recent years a political movement has targeted trans and non-binary children, and these efforts have already impacted the health and well-being of many young people and their families. The one positive possible outcome from this group's insistence that there isn't enough data about trans kids and medicine is that it could potentially help spur more high-quality studies. But remember that in states and countries where pubertal suppression isn't allowed for kids with gender dysphoria, it's still allowed and considered safe for cisgender kids with *precocious puberty* (early onset of puberty; you can find more info at https://www.mayoclinic.org/diseases-conditions/precocious-puberty/symptoms-causes/syc-20351811). The difference lies not in the safety of the treatment itself but in the reasons for prescribing it.

Beginning hormone therapy for children

Most young people use puberty-blocking drugs and take that time-out from natal puberty to work on discovering more about who they are and where their gender journey needs to go. For some, the answer to these questions is that they aren't trans after all, or that even though they are trans, they don't have gender dysphoria and don't want to undergo hormone treatment. This means coming off the puberty blockers and allowing natal puberty to begin, which is totally safe from a healthcare perspective.

Other kids definitely do want and need hormone therapy, and in these cases, their medical providers dovetail hormone treatment and puberty blockers. When to start hormone therapy is a complicated decision, but it's a decision for trans and non-binary kids and their families to make with the help and guidance of medical providers. For a lot of families, the perfect age is 13, so the child goes through only one puberty at the appropriate time, alongside the majority of their peers. No actual data or studies support a particular age as the "right" age to begin hormone treatment.

Chapter 9

Deciding to Undergo Surgery

M any trans and non-binary people laugh or possibly roll their eyes when cisgender people (whose gender and sex match) ask, "Have you had *the* surgery?" For a lot of trans folks, the answer to that question is another question: "Which one?" There are quite a few different surgeries that transgender and non-binary people can opt for. There are folks who want all, or nearly all, of the surgical procedures available, but there are also trans people who don't want to have any surgery (or can't for medical or other reasons).

In this chapter, we explore the world of gender-related surgeries. If you hear the phrase *transgender surgery* or *gender-affirming surgery,* and you only think of genital surgery, or possibly genital and chest surgeries, you aren't alone. It's a common misconception, so we're going to lay out detailed information about all the available options. For ease, this chapter is organized by masculinizing and feminizing surgeries, so check out both, or either, depending on what you're curious about.

Masculinizing Surgeries

If you're looking into masculinizing surgery, you'll discover a ton of information about the procedures often known as *top surgeries*. You may be surprised to find that there's more than one distinct surgical procedure you can undergo to create a flatter, more stereotypically masculine chest. You'll also discover that you can choose between three common genital surgeries: phalloplasty, metoidioplasty, and scrotoplasty.

Because there are so many surgeries you can opt into as part of a medical transition, you may find yourself a bit confused. In the following sections, we outline the procedures that are usually lumped together under masculinizing surgeries, starting with the most popular.

REMEMBER

Many trans masculine folks consider a hysterectomy part of their medical transition, although others don't want their uterus and ovaries removed. Some trans men want to be able to become pregnant and give birth, so for them, a hysterectomy is an unwanted and possibly emotionally painful experience. Others see the removal of their original *gonads* (internal reproductive organs) as something to celebrate. A hysterectomy (removal of the uterus) and oophorectomy (removal of the ovaries) stops the production of estrogen in the body, provides total protection against pregnancy, and guarantees that menstrual periods stop.

Top surgery

A 2022 article in the *International Journal of Transgender Health* (https://www.ncbi.nlm.nih.gov/pmc/articles/PMC9621289/) reported that of 298 people surveyed who identified as transgender men, 45 percent had undergone top surgery and 51 percent wanted it, with only 4 percent reporting that they weren't interested. For bottom surgery, the response was almost exactly the opposite: 4 percent had undergone some procedures, 50 percent were interested, and 46 percent said they weren't interested in pursuing bottom surgery.

As you can see from Figure 9-1, top surgery is the most popular surgical option for trans men and trans masculine folks.

REMEMBER

If this study doesn't reflect your goals and desires, that's absolutely fine. Gender journeys are personal, unique, and sometimes surprising!

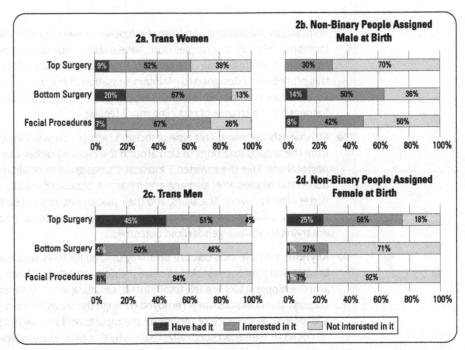

FIGURE 9-1: Results from a study about different transgender surgeries.

2a. Trans Women

	Have had it	Interested in it	Not interested in it
Top Surgery	9%	52%	39%
Bottom Surgery	20%	67%	13%
Facial Procedures	7%	67%	26%

2b. Non-Binary People Assigned Male at Birth

	Have had it	Interested in it	Not interested in it
Top Surgery	30%		70%
Bottom Surgery	14%	50%	36%
Facial Procedures	8%	42%	50%

2c. Trans Men

	Have had it	Interested in it	Not interested in it
Top Surgery	45%	51%	4%
Bottom Surgery	4%	50%	46%
Facial Procedures	6%	94%	

2d. Non-Binary People Assigned Female at Birth

	Have had it	Interested in it	Not interested in it
Top Surgery	25%	56%	18%
Bottom Surgery	1%	27%	71%
Facial Procedures	1% 7%		92%

Have had it — Interested in it — Not interested in it

Bita Tristani-Firouzi et al., 2021 /Taylor & Francis Group /https://pmc.ncbi.nlm.nih.gov/articles/PMC9621289/, last accessed on 15 January 2025.

Types of top surgeries

It's important to understand that top surgery for trans men isn't a one-size-fits-all surgery. Surgeons use several different types of *incisions* (surgical cuts) and procedures to remove the breasts and/or contour the chest when performing this gender-affirming operation. Folx Health has a great guide to top surgeries, with terrific illustrations of the incisions/scar sites at https://www.folxhealth.com/library/top-surgery-101-procedures-cost-and-safety. Here's a rundown of the various top surgeries you may consider:

>> **Double incision:** One of the most common versions of top surgery, double incision is a *bilateral mastectomy,* or removal of the breast tissue on both sides, through two incisions made along the *pectoral* (chest muscle) line. It can be done with or without nipple grafting and reconstruction. This means removing the nipples surgically, usually resizing them to a more typically masculine size, and then surgically reattaching them, often in a more *lateral* position (away from the middle, or toward the outside of your chest). Double incision is often the best choice for folks who have breasts larger than a typical B cup.

>> **Inverted T or anchor:** This is also a good option for folks who have large breasts but place a high priority on retaining as much feeling as possible. The incisions are made along the pectoral line as with a double incision, but

vertical cuts are made down from the nipples to meet up with the horizontal incisions. This way, the nipples don't have to be completely cut out and reattached. While any surgery can injure nerves and cause a loss of feeling, this procedure is designed to maintain sensation in the breasts. Because some tissue must be left under the nipple, you may sacrifice complete flatness for the chance of retaining more feeling.

>> **Fishmouth/batwing:** This type of incision radiates outward in both directions from the *areolas* (the rings of skin around the nipples) rather than along the pectoral line. Like the inverted T incision, it's designed to retain more sensation in the nipples after surgery, and it has the benefit of usually appearing flatter after recovery. The scars, and their placement, don't create a typically masculine-looking chest, so this option is sometimes favored by people who are trying to achieve genderfluid outcomes.

>> **Keyhole:** Keyhole incisions are primarily utilized for folks who have very small breasts and tighter chest skin. A small incision is made just below the areolas, and the nipple stalks are left totally intact, resulting in more sensation after surgery. The breast tissue is removed through the small incision, so there isn't a lot of leeway to resize or reposition the nipples and any excess skin can't be removed or tightened surgically. That's why this procedure is typically done with people who have A-cup (or smaller) breasts.

>> **Periareolar:** These incisions are also called *circumareolar* or *donut* surgeries. In this procedure for folks with small chests, one incision is made around the edge of each areola, and then another circular incision is made around the outside of the first incision, creating a "donut." The skin and the excess tissue are removed, and then the outside edge is pulled to the inside and closed up. This process leaves the nipple stalks intact and preserves sensation. The nipples can be downsized, but not repositioned, which is a drawback for some people, because it means that the nipples are in a more interior and higher position (a stereotypically feminine position).

>> **Buttonhole:** Buttonhole incisions, the last of the incisions that work better for people with small chests, are very similar to inverted T incisions. Imagine an inverted T and take away the vertical incision, and you have a buttonhole. The patient's smaller chest and tighter skin make the vertical incision unnecessary. The scar and nipple placement issues described in the other surgeries for people with small chests also occur with buttonhole incisions.

TIP

Some people don't want to have nipples at all. This can be more gender-affirming for folks, or just esthetically pleasing. Know that you can opt to have your nipples removed, or simply not reattached if you are having a procedure where they are removed.

REMEMBER

Some healthcare providers focus on your weight and *body mass index,* or *BMI* (a measurement of body fat based on your height and weight), when you're pursuing top surgery. However, many studies have shown that BMI is a bogus predictor of gender-affirming surgery outcomes. In fact, a 2023 Johns Hopkins study showed pretty conclusively that BMI is not at all a good indicator of who may experience serious complications with top surgery (https://tinyurl.com/24f935xe).

Recovering from top surgery

Postsurgical pain and scarring vary from person to person, so it's impossible to predict what your experience will be with either of those aspects of top surgery. Pain is very subjective, but the majority of patients who decide on top surgery report high levels of satisfaction and don't typically say that they regret their decision because of the pain they experienced. The different types of incisions can cause different amounts of severe or visible scarring, but you'll have some scarring even with the smaller incisions.

Scars are hard to predict, but you can do some things to help your scars heal well. It takes about 12 months for scars to fully mature so that you can essentially see what they'll look like. In that first year, you can protect your scars and help them heal by taking these steps:

>> **Keep them completely covered when you're in the sun.** If you can't do that, always use sunscreen.

>> **Massage them.** You can start rubbing and applying gentle pressure to the skin around your scars within the first four to six weeks after surgery.

>> **Listen to your surgeon!** They're going to tell you not to raise your arms over your head for at least three weeks and not to exercise for about that long. You'll have weight-lifting restrictions for at least six weeks. You may be impatient to get back to the gym, but these few weeks off are worthwhile compared to the ways you can make your scars worse by going against medical advice.

WARNING

It's important to recognize that some people lose grafted nipples. Most folks have good outcomes, but a small percentage experience graft failure, leaving them without nipples. Similarly, some people don't retain sensation in their nipples, despite all efforts to encourage this outcome. If you feel like top surgery is important for you, make sure you weigh how you'll feel if you have these outcomes.

Top surgery costs

In terms of cost, many transition-related surgeries are covered by insurance plans these days. This is really good news, but it comes with some barriers.

For example, many of the surgeons who work with transgender and non-binary people don't require letters from behavioral health professionals or psychiatrists before they perform different procedures, but some still do require those documents. And some surgeons don't accept health insurance or Medicaid, so you have to do your research to find out which providers accept your insurance.

Some folks opt to pay for top surgery out of pocket so that they can see whichever surgeon they want. You can find a list of many surgeons in the United States who perform top surgery at https://www.topsurgery.net and get an idea of the out-of-pocket costs some of them charge at https://www.topsurgery.net/costs/.

TIP

Don't be discouraged if a surgeon near you doesn't do the procedure you want. If your state doesn't have a surgeon who performs top surgery, or your insurance plan doesn't have an in-network provider, your insurer may be required to pay your expenses to see an out-of-network surgeon. But don't forget that you may have some out-of-pocket costs, even if your insurance pays for your travel and lodging while you're out of town having surgery (which they sometimes do.). The most important thing is to work with the surgeon's office to obtain preauthorization from your insurance company or to make a payment arrangement if you don't have insurance. Some surgeons have staff who are trained to help with this process.

Bottom surgery

Bottom surgery is a broad term that encompasses several gender-affirming surgical procedures to create a penis and/or scrotum and testicles and to remove female reproductive organs (you can find good info about these procedures and illustrations at https://us-uk.bookimed.com/article/female-to-male-bottom-surgery/). The three surgical options for constructing a penis and scrotum are

>> **Phalloplasty:** This is the creation of a penis (sometimes called a *neophallus*) and *urethra* (the tube that connects the bladder to the outside of the body so you can urinate) using tissue harvested from another part of the body. You have several different options for donor sites for the tissue used to create the penis (see the next section, "Types of phalloplasty").

>> **Metoidioplasty:** This surgery simply releases your own small penis from the ligament that restricts it. Especially if you take testosterone, you may see remarkable growth in the part of the vulva commonly called the *clitoris* (for information on masculinizing hormone therapy, go to Chapter 8). Many trans masculine people view this as their penis, referring to it with one of the many different words typically used for penis. This organ is limited in size and length by a suspensory ligament that's removed during surgery along with a fold of

connective tissue called the *labia minora*. You can find a good series of illustrations that clarifies the procedure at https://www.gender confirmation.com/bottom-surgery-ftm-metoidioplasty/.

>> **Scrotoplasty:** This optional procedure can be added to a phalloplasty or a metoidioplasty to create a scrotum and the appearance of testicles with silicone implants. The *labia majora* (fatty folds of the vulva) are used to hold the testicular implants and are surgically modified so they're in the correct position and connected to look like a typical scrotum. Sometimes tissue expanders are used to make room for the implants.

Types of phalloplasty

You can opt for different surgical procedures as part of a phalloplasty, but the main thing that distinguishes your phalloplasty options is where the graft is harvested on your body. Although at least six to eight different types of flaps can be utilized, some of the common ones are as follows:

>> **Groin flap:** As suggested by the name, this procedure uses tissue harvested from your groin/hip to create a larger penis (also called a *phallus*). It results in minimal visible scarring, but it creates a penis with about the same amount of touch sensation as any other part of your body. Some people say it creates a smaller penis than other procedures (like the forearm graft), but if you Google photos of completed surgeries, you can judge the size of the outcomes for yourself.

>> **Anterolateral thigh (ALT) flap:** This surgery uses a large flap of skin, fat, and connective tissue from the upper and outer part of your thigh. Because the donor site may be more visible when you're wearing shorts or swimming trunks, some patients are concerned about the size and appearance of the scar. ALT flap surgery creates a larger phallus, though, and allows for erotic sensation in the phallus, unlike groin flap surgery.

>> **Radial forearm flap (RFF):** RFF surgery, in which the donor flap is taken from your forearm, is currently the most common type of phalloplasty. The advantages and disadvantages are very similar to those of ALT surgery: a large visible scar (which is harder to cover up than a scar on the upper thigh), but erotic (or *erogenous*) sensation in the penis and typically a larger phallus.

>> **Musculocutaneous latissimus dorsi (MLD) flap:** For MLD surgery, the flap is harvested from your back or side. The latissimus dorsi muscle starts at the lower part of your spine, curves up around your side, and attaches to the upper bone of your arm. MLD surgery doesn't result in erotic sensation, but it typically creates a large penis and leaves a scar that's easily covered.

Some trans masculine people place a high priority on having a large penis. The complex mix of gender dysphoria and cultural influences that suggest that penis size is very important to potential sexual partners makes this understandable. Reading an article about that myth written for cisgender men who have sex with women may clarity the issue for you (https://www.hims.com/blog/what-size-penis-do-women-prefer). You can also check out photos of cisgender men's penises online. Even a casual scroll through an online gallery shows you the amazing variety of penises that cisgender men are born with (https://commons.wikimedia.org/wiki/Category:Close-up_photographs_of_human_penises).

To see the results of different types of phalloplasty, as well as metoidioplasty and glansplasty (which we cover in the later section "Related surgeries"), you can check out an online photo gallery from one surgeon in San Francisco (https://www.gurecon.com/photos). A lot of surgeons who perform these procedures share photos, either on their website or by request, and it's a great idea to look over the results from the surgeon(s) you're interested in. You can also check out YouTube for more information. One trans YouTuber makes videos in which he talks about many aspects of gender-affirming surgery and being a trans man (https://www.youtube.com/@Jammidodger). Of course, he represents just one perspective, his own, but it can be helpful to hear directly from other trans people.

Recovery and potential complications

Figure 9-2 shows the recovery times for trans masculine genital surgeries, including metaoidioplasty with urethral lengthening (see the later section "Related surgeries").

Time recommended	Meta w/Urethral Length	Phallo Flap – ALT	Phallo Flap – Groin	Phallo Flap – Radial Arm
In ICU or Equivalent	0	3 nights	3 nights	3 nights
In Hospital	2-3 nights	5-7 additional nights	5-7 additional nights	5-7 additional nights
In Town	2 additional weeks	3-4 additional weeks	3-4 additional weeks	3-4 additional weeks
Off Work	3-4 weeks	6 weeks – 3 months	6 weeks – 3 months	6 weeks – 3 months
Work Restrictions	1 month	6 months	6 months	6 months
Multi-Stage Procedure	2-3 stages	Minimum 3 stages Could be 3-5	Minimum 3 stages Could be 3-5	Minimum 3 stages Could be 3-5
Time between stages	3-5 months	3-5 months	3-5 months	3-5 months
In Home Care Needs	Phone support	Visiting Nursing or Support Person	Visiting Nursing or Support Person	Visiting Nursing or Support Person
Anticipated Complications	Extrusion of implants Implant Malposition	Flap Healing, Donor Site Healing, Stricture, Fistula	Flap Healing, Donor Site Healing, Stricture, Fistula	Flap Healing, Donor Site Healing, Stricture, Fistula
Total Time Possible	6 months	2 years	2 years	2 years

FIGURE 9-2:
Table of genital surgery recovery times.

Adapted from Bita Tristani-Firouzi et al., 2021, https://pmc.ncbi.nlm.nih.gov/articles/PMC9621289/, last accessed on 15 January 2025

Although phalloplasty is a great option for some trans and non-binary folks, it's also the masculinizing surgery covered in this section that is most likely to have complications. This list of complications isn't meant to discourage you, but to give you enough information to make your best decision. Some common issues that can arise with phalloplasty include the following:

>> **Bleeding/infection:** These complications can happen with virtually any surgery, but you should be aware of them.

>> **Complications from anesthesia:** These can include broken teeth from the insertion of the breathing tub or allergic reactions to the medicines.

>> **Flap failure:** Phalloplasty involves the grafting of a donor flap from one part of your body onto your groin to create a new penis. Anytime you do a graft, there's a possibility that the donor tissue will partially or totally fail to survive.

>> **Urethral fistulas:** You may develop a *fistula,* or small hole, in the new urethra that leaks urine. A lot of these spontaneously close, but some may have to be addressed surgically.

>> **Urethral strictures:** Sometimes scar tissue or hair growth in the new or lengthened urethra can cause a narrowing (or *stricture*) or even total blockage, making it difficult or impossible to pee. A *catheter* (small tube) may have to be inserted, or the urethra may even have to be repaired through further surgical procedures.

>> **Wound breakdown (also called *dehiscence*):** Sometimes the wound doesn't close normally or splits open and requires special care to close up.

Erections and orgasms post-surgery

You may be wondering, *What about sex?* Penetrative sex with your new penis is definitely possible. Although a penis created by phalloplasty will never be able to achieve a spontaneous erection, a lot of people opt for the implantation of an erectile device so that their new penis can get hard enough to penetrate a partner.

Two types of implants are currently available: an inflatable device with a small pump on one side of the scrotum, or a bendable rod. Even though additional complications are associated with implants, many folks are excited and happy to be able to use their new penis in a penetrative sexual way with a partner or partners.

Another issue many people are curious about is the ability to experience orgasms after genital surgery. Depending on where your donor flap comes from, you may have erotic sensation in your penis, which your surgeon can enhance with certain procedures that preserve sensation. Damage to nerves, or failure of nerves to regenerate, is another complication that can occur with any surgery, but barring that, orgasm after a phalloplasty is possible.

Also, *clitoral burial* (putting the clitoral tissue under the base of the newly constructed penis) is an option to increase your orgasmic ability. That way, stimulation to the penis stimulates that erogenous tissue at the base of your penis.

Many trans masculine and non-binary people enjoy vaginal sex and orgasms. *Vaginectomy*, or the removal of the vaginal canal and closure of the vaginal opening, is one of the bottom surgery options. If you don't choose to have a vaginectomy, you'll still have a vaginal canal that you can utilize sexually.

Related surgeries

A handful of other procedures can be done in combination with a phalloplasty or metoidioplasty. Besides those covered in previous sections — erectile device implantation, scrotoplasty, and vaginectomy — the most common of these optional surgeries are

>> **Glansplasty:** This is the surgical creation of the *glans,* or head of the penis. The penis constructed by a phalloplasty won't naturally have a mushroom-shaped head, so it has to be surgically added. An incision is made around the phallus a few centimeters from the tip which creates a flap of skin that can be folded in and stitched. It is possible to do this in the first stage of a phallo, but it's most commonly done in stage 2.

>> **Mons resection:** This surgery combines the removal of skin with *liposuction* (fat removal) to reduce the often fatty, padded *mons,* or upper pubic area. Removing some fat and skin from this area can result in more forward placement and larger appearance of the phallus.

>> **Urethral lengthening:** This procedure stretches the urethra so it goes all the way to the tip of the penis, which allows most patients to stand to pee with their new penis. This is the one thing some guys have been wanting and waiting to do!

The final surgical procedures considered part of bottom surgery for trans masculine folks are hysterectomies and oophorectomies. Having a *hysterectomy* (surgical removal of the uterus) isn't a prerequisite for any of the other procedures, but some folks find it highly desirable. A hysterectomy can be done hand in hand with an *oophorectomy*, or surgical removal of the ovaries.

For transgender men and non-binary people who want to become pregnant and give birth, a hysterectomy or oophorectomy isn't a voluntary part of their transition-related care. But other people may opt for either or both procedures in order to guarantee the complete stoppage of periods, put up a total barrier to pregnancy from sexual activity, and eliminate the need for reproductive cancer screenings or any worry about future occurrence of reproductive cancer. If the possibility of pregnancy is a big concern for you, or causes you dysphoria, you can opt for a *tubal ligation* (surgically clipping or cauterizing the fallopian tubes) or contraception.

Bottom surgery costs

People choose one bottom surgery option over another for varying personal reasons and considerations. Sometimes these choices dovetail with your choice of a surgeon. We hope that trans and non-binary people will someday be able to choose the surgeon and procedure they want based only on personal reasons, and not be limited by finances.

Unfortunately, today isn't that day. If you have to utilize your health insurance to pay for your bottom surgery, you need to make sure your policy covers the procedure you want, and then find a surgeon who both performs that procedure and takes your insurance. Some surgeons have staff whose job is to help you navigate the world of deductibles and copays, so try not to be too intimidated.

TIP

Also, a whole lot of folks have successfully appealed initial denials and have gotten their bottom surgery covered, so if the insurer tries to deny you, appeal! It can seem difficult, so ask your healthcare provider if they can help. A list of surgeons on TransHealthCare.org who perform surgery for trans and non-binary people may be a good place to start (https://www.transhealthcare.org). You can search by surgical procedure, state, or even insurance type. Don't forget that you may need one or two letters from other healthcare providers to clear the red tape, especially if your insurance requires it.

Pondering Feminizing Surgeries

As with masculinizing surgeries, people seeking a medical transition can opt for a variety of feminizing surgeries. In the following sections, we outline the procedures that are usually lumped together under feminizing surgeries, starting with the face and then moving to top and bottom surgeries.

Facial feminization surgery

Facial feminization surgery (FFS) sounds like a single surgery, but it's actually a set of surgical procedures that are used in different combinations to reduce what are thought of as more typically masculine facial features and shape them into more stereotypically feminine features.

As with all transition-related surgeries, there are different levels of interest and need for this surgical option. For some trans feminine and non-binary people, FFS is the single most important step they will take, and surgically changing the shape and contours of their face makes them feel more like themself and healed than anything else. For others, FFS may not even be on the radar, or they may feel great about the way their face already looks. Watching a short video of a plastic surgeon explaining some aspects of FFS (https://www.plasticsurgery.org/video-gallery/facial-feminization-surgery) can help you understand the procedures.

While masculinizing face surgeries are something you may be hearing a little more about in 2024, testosterone therapy alone can change your face, not just spurring facial hair growth, but even reshaping your jawline and other facial features to varying degrees, depending on your genetics. For details about masculinizing hormone therapy, flip to Chapter 8.

FFS procedures

Each person's face is different, so whether you need (or want) any element of FFS really depends on your face type and your personal goals for surgery. The different facial features that can be altered by FFS include the following:

» **Adam's apple:** This procedure, called a tracheal shave, is just, as its name suggests, a shaving down of the cartilage that forms your Adam's apple, creating a flatter throat profile.

» **Brows:** A prominent brow can be associated with a male face, so the bones under your eyebrows, called the supraorbital ridge, can be shaved down as well.

» **Cheeks:** Like all FFS elements, the need for cheek surgery varies from person to person, but in some cases, a surgeon will perform cheekbone implants or reposition your cheekbones.

» **Chin:** A surgeon can lower the height of your chin, resulting in a more rounded appearance.

» **Forehead:** A common element of FFS is reducing the forehead, mainly by bringing your hairline down closer to your eyebrows and feminizing its shape on your forehead.

» **Jaw:** The pieces of FFS can sound scary, and jaw surgery is no exception. A surgeon often must saw part of your jawbone off to create a more rounded jawline.

» **Lips:** Reducing the space between the bottom of your nose and your upper lip can change the way your face is perceived. Fuller lips are also sometimes associated with a more feminine appearance, so lip filler may be part of your approach.

>> **Nose:** The size and shape of your nose can create a more stereotypically masculineor feminine-looking face, so rhinoplasty (or nose surgery) can be part of FFS as well.

Potential FFS complications

Complications from FFS can include

>> **Hematoma:** This buildup of blood under the skin is usually temporary.

>> **Permanent nerve damage:** It is possible to sever nerves during surgery, which can result in a loss of feeling, or even voluntary movement in areas of your face.

>> **Typical surgical complications:** These are mainly infection, bleeding, and complications from anesthesia.

>> **Wound breakdown (also called *dehiscence*):** The surgical wound may burst open or not close properly, and repairing it may require special care.

Top surgery

Top surgery for trans feminine people means one thing: breast augmentation. While a good number of people get the breast growth they want from feminizing hormone treatment (see Chapter 8), others don't. Either they don't want to take hormones but still want breasts, or they do want to take hormones but their genetic limitations on breast growth don't meet their wants and needs.

In these cases, trans women and non-binary people just seek out the same type of breast-enlarging surgery that cisgender women have been undergoing since at least the 1970s. This means either getting silicone (or saline) implants or transplanting fat from other parts of your body to create bigger breasts. If you're going to take feminizing hormones, most surgeons recommend that you be on estrogen for at least one year to see what type of breast growth you may be able to achieve from that alone before moving on to surgery.

Bottom surgery

Lower, or bottom, surgeries for trans feminine folks include vaginoplasty, vulvo-plasty, and orchiectomy. *Vaginoplasty* is the creation of a *vagina* (the internal canal leading to the uterus in cisgender women), and *vulvoplasty* is the creation of a *vulva* (the external female genitals) without a vaginal canal. *Orchiectomy* is simply the surgical term for the removal of the testicles. You can find a list of some surgeons around the world who perform bottom surgery at https://www.transhealthcare.org/.

Wanting to preserve your penis doesn't make you any less of a woman or any less trans. Many trans women and non-binary people love their penis and enjoy using it sexually. It's absolutely possible to have a vulvoplasty that leaves your penis intact, without having a vaginoplasty. Talk to your surgeon if this sounds like something that interests you.

You can search online for feminizing surgeries by surgical procedure, state, or even insurance type. Some surgeons share pictures of their results on their website (for example, you can see terrific pictures of one surgeon's vaginoplasties at https://cranects.com/vaginoplasty-photos/). Many surgeons have photos of their results, even if they don't post them on their website. If you're interested in working with a specific surgeon, ask to see photos of their previous patients.

Types of bottom surgeries

Because testosterone is so powerful that folks who still have their testes must block it, testicle removal can be a great relief to some people. Not only can they get rid of the *antiandrogen* (testosterone-blocking) portion of their hormone therapy regimen, but people who've had an orchiectomy also report a general feeling of well-being from not having gonads pumping testosterone into their body anymore.

An orchiectomy is a very simple procedure, and even though general anesthesia is used, it often takes only about 30 minutes to complete. Complications and recovery time are minimal. The scrotal tissue can be removed at the same time, which is called a *scrotectomy*. However, if you think that you may want a vaginoplasty or vulvoplasty, this isn't advised, because the scrotal tissue is used to construct the vulva.

An orchiectomy can be performed on its own, but it's definitely one of the steps in a vaginoplasty. Although a vaginoplasty is significantly more complicated, many trans feminine people feel very strongly about undergoing this surgery. *Penile inversion vaginoplasty*, the most common procedure, essentially involves inverting, or turning inside out, the existing penile skin to create the vaginal canal. Some of the erectile tissue from the removed penis is used to create a clitoris during a vulvoplasty.

The surgeon performing a vaginoplasty doesn't create a mucus membrane, so the vaginal canal doesn't self-lubricate. Some procedures address this by, for example, bringing part of the abdominal lining, or *peritoneum*, into the vaginal canal to line it. There are several possible steps to a vaginoplasty, and some can be undertaken on their own.

REMEMBER

If you haven't seen a whole lot of cisgender women's vulvas, you may be under the mistaken impression that they all look alike. That's definitely not true. Folks' genitals look as different as their faces do. You should absolutely come out of your transition process with the highest level of satisfaction, but try not to buy into the myth of the "ideal" woman. Cisgender women run the gamut of size, shape, and appearance, and so do trans women. You are beautiful!

Other procedures you may want or need include

>> **Labiaplasty:** This procedure isn't required, but many people feel like their results are better if they include this step as part of their feminizing surgery. During a labiaplasty, the scrotal tissue is used to make the labia majora, labia minora, and clitoral hood. See Figure 9-3 for a simple illustration of this anatomy.

>> **Permanent hair removal:** Especially if you're going the penile inversion route, you'll most likely have to do electrolysis or laser hair removal on and around the penis and scrotum. Hair growing in the new vaginal canal may cause infections or even pain during penetrative sex.

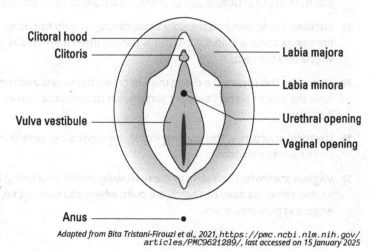

FIGURE 9-3:
An illustration of the parts of a vulva.

Clitoral hood
Clitoris
Labia majora
Labia minora
Vulva vestibule
Urethral opening
Vaginal opening
Anus

Adapted from Bita Tristani-Firouzi et al., 2021, https://pmc.ncbi.nlm.nih.gov/ articles/PMC9621289/, last accessed on 15 January 2025

WARNING

Before having bottom surgery, you may have to get letters from a counselor, a psychiatrist, and/or a primary care doctor. While this is often an excessive amount of jumping through hoops to get your surgery, your insurance may require it in order to cover your procedure(s).

Recovering and possible complications

Depending on which procedures you're having, bottom surgery can take several hours, and may even be done in two stages months apart. You may be in the hospital for a few days, and you'll have several weeks of recovery. After that, you enter into a lifelong commitment of doing something called *dilation* (inserting an object into the vaginal canal to keep it open and flexible).

You usually dilate your vaginal canal frequently (four times per day) in the first month after surgery, then a little less often for the next 5 months (two times per day), and then once a day for months 6–12 post-surgery. While you'll have to dilate for the rest of your life, the frequency varies from person to person. Some folks may do it only once a month.

Complications from bottom surgery can range from minor to pretty serious. They include

>> **Bleeding/infection:** These are the most common complications for any kind of surgery, so you should be aware of them.

>> **Complications from anesthesia:** These can include broken teeth from the insertion of the breathing tub or allergic reactions to the medicines.

>> **Fistulas:** These holes accidentally made during surgery can occur between the vagina and the bladder, but this is less common than fistulas between the vagina and the rectum.

>> **Necrosis:** This means the tissue used to create the vagina and vulva may not have the proper blood flow after surgery, which can cause part or all of it to die.

>> **Urethral strictures:** This scarring inside the urethra can restrict the flow of urine from the bladder.

>> **Vaginal stenosis:** This refers to the narrowing and/or shortening of the vaginal canal. Stenosis can reach the point where you may not be able to engage in penetrative sex.

REMEMBER

Speaking of sex, you may be wondering if you can have sex after bottom surgery and what it will feel like. Most folks who have feminizing surgery are able to enjoy their new body and have orgasms. Your healthcare provider will recommend that you wait at least three months after vaginoplasty to have penetrative sex. It can take months for the swelling to go down completely and for you to figure out how sex feels now. Try to be patient with yourself and have fun. Pelvic floor physical therapy can be an effective way to keep your new vagina healthy and happy.

An article published in the *International Journal of Transgender Health* (https://www.ncbi.nlm.nih.gov/pmc/articles/PMC9621289/) gives you an idea about how folks relate to gender-affirming surgeries. Figure 9-4 lists some common barriers to surgeries for trans and non-binary people, and Figure 9-5 shines a light on the reasons some people aren't interested in these surgical procedures. As always, others' experiences don't need to match up with your experience. Everyone is on their own journey.

Feminizing surgery costs

In terms of cost, many transition-related surgeries are covered by insurance plans these days. This is really exciting, but it comes with some barriers.

Many surgeons who work with transgender and non-binary people don't require letters from behavioral health professionals or psychiatrists before they perform gender-affirming procedures, but some still do require those documents. And some surgeons don't accept health insurance or Medicaid, so you have to do your research to find out which providers accept your insurance. Some folks opt to pay for surgery out of pocket so they can see whichever surgeon they want.

TIP

If your state doesn't have a surgeon who performs the procedure(s) you want, or your insurance plan doesn't include an in-network provider, your insurer may be required to pay your expenses to see an out-of-network surgeon. Don't be discouraged if a surgeon near you doesn't do the surgery you're looking for.

But don't forget that you may have some out-of-pocket costs, even if your insurance pays for your travel and lodging while you're out of town having surgery (which they sometimes do.). The most important thing is to work with the surgeon's office to obtain preauthorization for your surgery or to make a payment arrangement if you don't have insurance. Some surgeons have staff who are trained to help with this process.

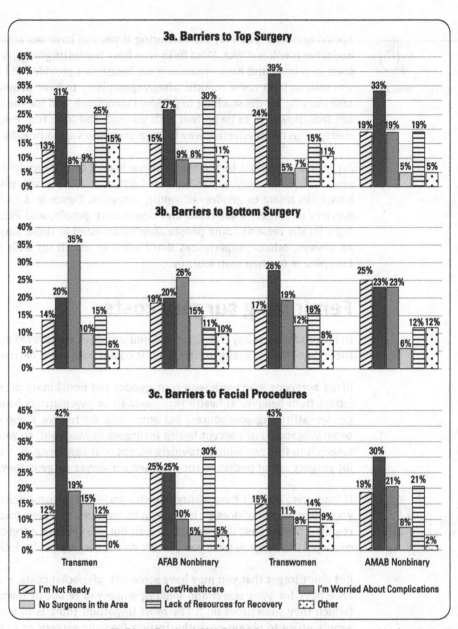

3a. Barriers to Top Surgery

3b. Barriers to Bottom Surgery

3c. Barriers to Facial Procedures

Legend:
- I'm Not Ready
- Cost/Healthcare
- I'm Worried About Complications
- No Surgeons in the Area
- Lack of Resources for Recovery
- Other

X-axis categories: Transmen, AFAB Nonbinary, Transwomen, AMAB Nonbinary

FIGURE 9-4: Common barriers to gender-affirming surgeries.

Bita Tristani-Firouzi et al., 2021 /Taylor & Francis Group / https://pmc.ncbi.nlm.nih.gov/ articles/PMC9621289/, last accessed on 15 January 2025

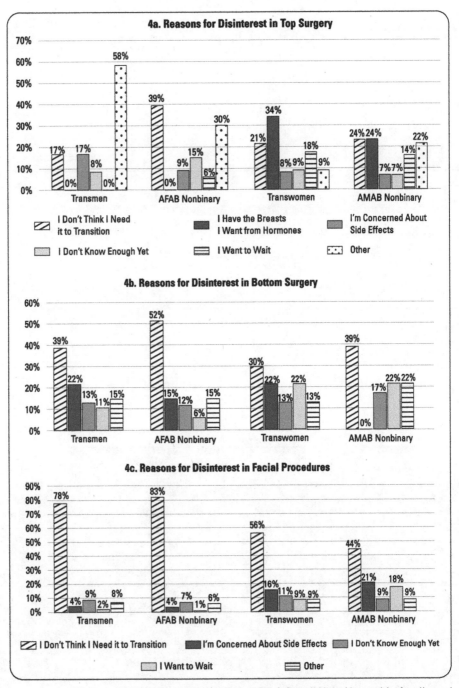

FIGURE 9-5: Reasons for disinterest in gender-affirming surgeries.

Bita Tristani-Firouzi et al., 2021 /Taylor & Francis Group /https://pmc.ncbi.nlm.nih.gov/articles/PMC9621289/, last accessed on 15 January 2025

IN THIS CHAPTER

» **Finding your voice with speech training**

» **Feminizing or masculinizing your voice**

» **Considering voice surgery options**

Chapter **10**

Changing Your Tune with Voice and Speech Therapy

For some transgender and non-binary people, masculinizing or feminizing their voice is a crucial step in their transition. People have reported that they have much more confidence, openness to interacting with others, and willingness to put themselves out into the world after undergoing voice training or speech therapy or even surgical procedures to change their voice.

In this chapter, you get an overview of some options for changing your voice. Vocal changes for trans folks mostly center around speech therapy and voice training, but a few surgical possibilities also exist.

REMEMBER

The decision to change the sound of your voice is like all the other gender-affirming options we outline in this book. It's deeply personal, and doesn't validate or invalidate your gender or your transgender or non-binary status. Some trans people feel supremely confident using their natural voice and can't imagine making any effort to change the way they speak. Your feelings about your voice are part of your gender journey and shouldn't be used to judge you or where you are on that journey. If you aren't thrilled with how your voice sounds at this moment, read on. You really can do some things to significantly change your voice and the way it's perceived by others.

Talking about Voice Training

Current research and scientific thought strongly support the concept that human beings are essentially "wired" for connection and attachment. You can read about this idea and much more in the work of Gabor Maté, Johann Hari, Bruce Alexander, and others. So, connection and relationships are important for humans, and communication is one of the primary ways people engage in relationships with others. This is why it feels so important to be truly heard and recognized as your correct gender when you communicate.

Strategies for changing the way you speak often focus on specific vocal techniques designed to help train your voice. Each of the qualities below can impact others' perception of your voice as more stereotypically masculine or feminine.

Working with a vocal coach or speech therapist raises your awareness of the following speech and vocal characteristics that can impact the way others hear your voice:

>> **Articulation:** This involves the careful enunciation of sounds and syllables to ensure that speech is understood.

   In other words, it's the clarity and precision with which sounds and words are formed.

>> **Frequency:** This refers to the number of times the vocal cords vibrate, which affects *pitch,* or how high or low a voice sounds.

   Higher frequencies are often associated with feminine-sounding voices, and lower frequencies are typically linked to masculine voices.

>> **Inflection:** This refers to changes in the voice during speech. In addition to the volume of a speaker's voice, inflection includes factors like tone or pitch going up or down at the end of a sentence.

>> **Intensity:** This involves the volume of a speaker's voice as well as the force and speed with which they speak.

>> **Resonance:** This characteristic results from the way sound vibrates in the vocal tract.

   Resonance affects the depth and richness of a voice. A voice with more resonance may sound fuller or more rounded; less resonance can make the voice sound thinner or nasal.

>> **Vocal quality:** This refers to the amount of breath in someone's speaking voice.

>> **Weight:** This describes whether a voice is perceived as "light" or "heavy." Lighter voices are sometimes described as bright, and heavier voices may be characterized as rich, or powerful.

Lots of these vocal characteristics are reflections of the vibration of the vocal cords or the way the air passed through the vocal tract.

An image from the Cleveland Clinic in Figure 10-1 gives a simple overview of the vocal cords and where they're located.

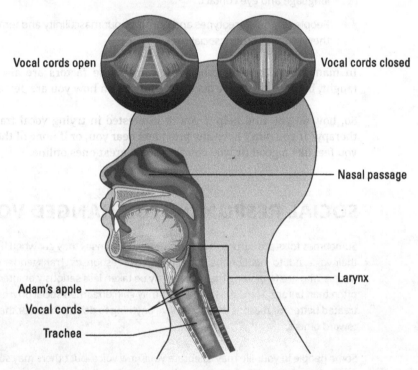

Vocal cords open

Vocal cords closed

Nasal passage

Larynx

Adam's apple

Vocal cords

Trachea

FIGURE 10-1:
An illustration of
the vocal cords.

Other factors that influence how people interpret (and assign gender to) your voice may include

>> **Age:** Society often has different expectations for how people of different genders sound at different stages of life.

>> **Cultural factors:** Masculine and feminine stereotypes change dramatically from one cultural group to another, and even within a single culture over time.

>> **Paraverbal keys:** Nonverbal cues like facial expressions, posture, and hand gestures can affect the way people are perceived.

This can also include factors like amount of lip movement and mouth openness.

>> **Region:** If you think about the United States, for example, you may understand how differences in gender norms and stereotypes, even subtle ones, from one region to another can affect perceptions about someone's voice.

>> **Social cues:** These are related to paraverbal keys and include things like body language and eye contact.

People rely on stereotypes and norms about masculinity and femininity when they interpret others' social cues.

In many vocal training programs, some these factors are also examined and taught, because they have such a big impact on how you are perceived socially.

So, how do you find help if you're interested in trying vocal training or speech therapy? If you don't have any providers near you, or if none of the providers near you feel like a good fit, you can find some great ones online.

SOCIAL RESPONSES TO CHANGED VOICES

Sometimes folks are surprised at the different responses they get when they change their voice, not to mention the intensity of those responses. Transgender women, or people who are feminizing their voice, may be taken less seriously or interrupted more often than before. Trans masculine folks may gain unearned social privilege — being treated better for reasons that don't have anything to do with them or their behavior toward others.

Some people in your life may celebrate your new voice, but others may struggle to accept it or may even express some doubt or dislike of the way you speak and communicate now.

As with many elements of gender transition, changing your voice can be a roller-coaster! Expect to have some days when you feel more confident about the way you come across and others when you feel more insecure, and to have ups and downs when the people in your life acknowledge, accept, or have difficulties with your new voice.

Although they don't take insurance at this time, Seattle Voice Lab provides online services (https://www.seattlevoicelab.com). Connected Speech Pathology is another online provider that offers voice training (https://connectedspeech pathology.com). Google "gender-affirming speech therapy" or "gender-affirming voice training" and see what you come up with.

The World Professional Association for Transgender Health offers a provider search tool that can help you find in-person services in a lot of different specialties, including vocal therapy (https://www.wpath.org/provider/search).

The American Speech-Language-Hearing Association also has a good search tool called ProFind that allows you to select Transgender Voice as a specific area of expertise (https://tinyurl.com/yuk2hx3a).

WARNING

Some providers in the speech-language pathology field feel strongly that trans and non-binary people should use self-guided voice training only under professional supervision. Because each person, and their voice, is different, you may experience vocal fatigue or changes that are the opposite of what you're going for if you start a self-guided online program completely on your own.

A good way to keep that from happening is to have at least an initial consultation and assessment with a professional. Then you'll have that person as a resource in the future, along with your primary healthcare provider, if you have any issues with your self-guided vocal training program.

A great provider will offer services that are client-centered and available to people of all genders and gender expressions. The other choices you make about your transition and gender-affirming treatments shouldn't limit your access to voice training, and neither should any disability or difference you have. Vocal training services can be adapted in many ways, so hold out for a provider who knows how to work with you and accommodate your individual needs. In the end there's only one way to evaluate the results of a voice training program: your satisfaction with your voice!

REMEMBER

Although some providers of gender voice therapy don't accept insurance, and some insurance plans don't cover it, you should check to see if yours does. Even Medicaid plans pay for this type of gender-affirming treatment in some places.

According to a KFF (formerly known as the Kaiser Family Foundation) survey from 2022 about Medicaid coverage of different transition-related treatments (https://tinyurl.com/3x8v6cvt), "Thirteen of the 41 responding survey states report that they cover gender-affirming speech or voice therapy services, some requiring prior authorization. Ten of the survey states reported that they exclude coverage for gender-affirming voice therapy services, and 18 states responded that they have not addressed this coverage in their state policy."

VOICE TRAINING WITH CHILDREN

People often wonder whether kids can do voice training, and the answer is yes! You have to find a therapist or provider who has expertise and experience with children, but there's no reason young trans and non-binary people can't start working on their voice as early as 11 or 12.

If young people have to go through their natal puberty — in other words, if they don't have access to puberty blockers — voice training can help lessen the gender dysphoria (distress over the mismatch between their gender and assigned sex) the "wrong" voice may be starting to cause.

Finding Your Gendered Voice

You can train your voice to sound more stereotypically feminine or masculine, or you can train your voice to sound *androgynous* (having both masculine and feminine characteristics). If you're curious or skeptical about the results of voice training, you can listen to recordings of all three types of students on Seattle Voice Lab's website (https://www.seattlevoicelab.com/testimonials/), and you can find many other examples of gender-affirming speech therapy on the internet.

REMEMBER

The voice you start your vocal training with is a product of your culture and upbringing, but it's also a product of your genetics. Cisgender men can have very high voices, and cisgender women can have very low ones. Remember this if you decide that vocal training or therapy isn't for you.

Going for a feminine voice

Hormones can play a part in both the masculinizing and feminizing of voices. For transgender women, the biggest issue is the effect of the testosterone that changed their voices during natal puberty.

REMEMBER

If you were able to take puberty blockers, then testosterone didn't deepen your voice during your teens. But many trans feminine people are trying to feminize their voice because it was lowered by testosterone-based natal puberty. A lower-pitched voice is one of the few truly irreversible effects of testosterone (other than hair loss and, for some people, hair growth). Unfortunately, if you opt to take feminizing hormones, they won't have any impact on your voice.

Although there are lots of different ideas about how to best achieve the results you want, one basic premise to keep in mind is that a more masculine voice comes from pushing your sound and air down toward the *larynx* (the part of the throat where the vocal cords are), while a more feminine voice comes from up in the cheekbones.

You can get an idea of what to expect during feminizing voice training by checking out different providers' websites. For example, Gender Voice SLP in New Mexico gives an overview of their methods at `https://www.gendervoiceslp.com/curriculum`, and Seattle Voice Lab provides helpful information about their voice feminizing program at `https://www.seattlevoicelab.com/services/male-to-female-voice/`.

TIP

No matter which type of voice training you choose, it's important to take good care of yourself during therapy. Gender Voice SLP recommends "vocal rest for at least four hours after session (no talking, no practice); throat lozenges; water; warm tea; Throat Coat tea. Sleep!" as great ways to preserve the voice you're working to obtain. Other helpful advice is to practice, although not too much, and to record yourself and listen to your voice to get a clearer sense of how you sound.

WARNING

One concern specific to trans women's gender-affirming care is the (very rare) complication that tracheal shave surgery, which reduces the appearance of the Adam's apple, can harm the vocal folds. Going to a skilled surgeon should minimize or eliminate your risk. Another infrequent voice-related complication from this surgery is *laryngospasm* (muscle spasms of the vocal cords). This condition usually resolves within a week.

Working to masculinize your voice

Trans men starting hormone therapy often focus on the following concerns about their voice:

» How soon will voice changes be noticeable?

» How low will their frequency or pitch get?

» How long will it take to reach their masculine voice and become permanent?

» How will their singing voice be affected?

Vocal outcomes vary from person to person, so those questions are difficult to answer. Hormone therapy can definitely play a big part in changing your voice, and many people who are trying to masculinize their voice find that taking testosterone, or T, is one of the most effective ways to do it.

But because of genetics and other factors, some people aren't satisfied with the vocal outcomes they get from T alone for the following reasons:

» **They've had little to no lowering of vocal frequency and pitch after a year on hormones.** This can be evidence of some type of hormonal or physiological issue. At the one-year mark of hormone therapy, patients on T should be checking in with their primary healthcare provider, who can diagnose and treat some of these issues. An endocrinologist may also be able to help.

» **They have access to stereotypically male vocal frequencies but don't consistently speak at them.** This issue may simply be a matter of retraining the vocal mechanisms and brain to utilize the new frequencies and pitch created by masculinizing hormones.

For people on T who aren't happy with their vocal changes and others who aren't interested in taking masculinizing hormones, vocal training or therapy can be the next step.

REMEMBER

It's important to know that you don't have to take hormones at all when you do vocal training. The techniques you pick up in therapy can help you craft a voice that feels more representative of your gender and the way you want to be perceived, even if you think hormones may never be part of your journey.

How does masculinizing your voice with vocal training work? As with feminizing speech therapy, there are many different approaches to achieving the voice you want, but one basic premise is that a more masculine voice comes from pushing your sound and air down toward your larynx, while a more feminine voice comes from up in the cheekbones. To get an idea of what therapy focuses on, check out some of the vocal training methods used by Gender Voice SLP (https://www.gendervoiceslp.com/curriculum) and Seattle Voice Lab (https://www.seattlevoicelab.com/services/female-to-male-voice/).

WARNING

Trans masculine folks who go through two cycles of puberty — the one attached to their designated sex at birth and their second puberty brought on by hormone therapy — should be aware of an important physical consideration. Cisgender men (whose gender and sex match) have longer vocal folds than cisgender women. A cisgender boy's vocal folds develop and reach the typical length associated with a masculine-sounding voice during their testosterone-based puberty. If you went through a "female" puberty as a teenager, your vocal folds didn't develop through this lengthening process, and they're unable to do it now. However, your vocal cords will thicken if you take T.

This situation can lead to a voice with a distinctive sound, sometimes described as almost robotic, that some guys don't like. Gradually increasing your T dose in the beginning (rather than initiating hormones at the full dose) can be a great way to prevent this effect, although it can be hard to be patient about other changes you've been anticipating. Voice training or therapy is a really good investment in a long-term voice you love.

Choosing neutral voice training

You may be interested in developing one consistent way of talking that falls between stereotypical masculine and feminine vocal registers and patterns, or you may want (or need) to develop both types of speaking voices to use at different times. In that case, vocal training and speech therapy can help you find a neutral or androgynous voice.

As with many aspects of being non-binary and challenging the gender binary, the idea of developing both a masculine and feminine way of speaking was controversial in the past, and speech professionals discouraged it. The thinking was that trying to speak in a neutral voice could strain your vocal cords or prevent you from practicing and developing one strong vocal presentation.

Although some people's internal gender matches best with having options for the way they speak, others may not be able to live openly as their true gender and need flexibility in their vocal communication. Fortunately, many voice therapists offer androgynous vocal training today.

SINGING AFTER A VOICE CHANGE

A significant number of trans people are interested in being able to sing during and after transition. The good news is, you can! In fact, many trans people love figuring out how to sing in a voice that matches their gender inside.

A gender voice coach or therapist can help you develop your singing voice on its own or as you're working on your new speaking voice. You can find out more in some good online articles about trans feminine and non-binary singing (https://tinyurl.com/3a2jere7) and trans masculine singing (https://tinyurl.com/y96jdk28).

Looking at Vocal Surgeries

The reviews and opinions of surgery for changing vocal pitch are mixed. A quick internet search yields a lot of different patient satisfaction statistics and stories. Some of the reported complications from voice surgeries, like infection and scarring, are common to most surgical procedures.

Other complications are specific to surgery involving your throat and voice, such as issues with vocal volume or quality, or restrictions on breathing or swallowing.

Although changing your voice through coaching and therapy can potentially cause significant strain, and surgery has the possibility to produce the desired changes without this strain, some professionals say that the possible complications don't outweigh this benefit.

If surgery is something you're considering, we recommend doing lots of research on the procedure you're interested in. If possible, talk to some of your doctor's other patients who've had the same surgery.

You can choose from several different types of surgery, including these common procedures:

>> **Cricothyroid approximation:** This feminizing surgery raises the tension on the vocal folds, creating a higher pitch. A common complaint from people who've had the procedure is that the results don't last.

>> **Feminization laryngoplasty:** This relatively new surgery changes the pitch and resonance of the voice as well as the appearance of the throat (by minimizing the Adam's apple, or thyroid cartilage).

>> **Medialization laryngoplasty (formerly called thyroplasty):** In the rare cases that trans men undergo voice-changing surgery, this is the procedure that masculinizes the voice.

>> **Wendler glottoplasty:** In this procedure, which is the most common voice-feminizing surgery, parts of the vocal cords are sewn together to shorten them and raise the voice's pitch.

REMEMBER

Some speech therapists who work with trans people tell stories of patients who came to voice training after having surgery because they were dissatisfied with the results. Although many patients are very happy with their surgical outcome, undergoing medical treatment that doesn't achieve your desired goal is always frustrating. But it's nice to know that voice training may still get you close to where you want to be if you either don't want to undergo surgery or don't feel completely satisfied with your surgical results.

Chapter **11**

Planning a Family

Transgender and non-binary people relate to the idea of biologically reproducing in various ways, which is another reason it's so important to remember that your journey is your own.

You have many different options for creating a family, and despite what you may have been told when you were growing up, or what the family you grew up with may believe, your family is real and valid in whatever way you make it.

Between the four people on the writing team, we have two folks who are child-free but who are major pet parents. And we have two who are parents, but neither have any genetic tissue in common with their kids.

REMEMBER

It's 100 percent okay — in fact, it's an admirable decision — to not have kids if that isn't something you feel a strong pull to do. The mainstream U.S. culture exerts a lot of pressure on people to become parents, and there are strong implicit and explicit biases about biological parenting. For many trans and queer families, having kids is expensive and takes extensive planning. It's an important and life-altering step, and it certainly isn't for everyone.

In this chapter, you discover a lot of the information you need to make very personal decisions about family planning and contraception. You also uncover information about fertility and the possible effects of medical transition on fertility. You may be surprised to find out that some common wisdom about this may be wrong!

Considering Your Options
if Planning a Family

It isn't for everyone, but having children from your genetic tissue may be really important to you. You can plan ahead to harvest and preserve your sperm or eggs before you begin your medical transition. Possible changes to fertility are discussed in the next section of this chapter (see "Understanding How Transition Care Can Impact Your Fertility"), but if you're just beginning to think about all this, rest assured that you do have some options.

Preserving genetic tissue

The retrieval and preservation of eggs is one of the options for transgender men, trans masculine folks, or non-binary people who were designated female at birth. This process is also called *oocyte cryopreservation*, which is just fancy talk for freezing eggs. There isn't a ton of data so far, but some initial findings suggest that you can have good results harvesting your eggs even after you have started testosterone.

WARNING

Egg retrieval does require you to discontinue taking testosterone, or T, possibly for a few months, and some folks find this to be very difficult. Also, experts have varying opinions about whether the viability of eggs *can* be affected by testosterone use, so many healthcare providers recommend that you undergo the harvesting process before you begin hormone therapy, if you haven't already started it. And keep in mind that oocyte cryopreservation is quite expensive.

The only transition option that makes egg retrieval truly impossible is the removal of the ovaries — the part of the body that makes and stores eggs. Here are the basic steps involved in egg retrieval and preservation:

>> **Hormone injections to stimulate the ovaries:** This matures or ripens the eggs, and it leads to elevated levels of estrogen in the blood.

   Along with not being able to take testosterone, this is another part of the process that can increase *gender dysphoria,* or feelings of gender misalignment, for some people.

>> **Transvaginal oocyte retrieval (TVOR):** When performing TVOR, your healthcare provider uses ultrasound to guide a large needle into the ovary to retrieve the eggs.

   You will be sedated for this, and it's usually done quickly.

- >> **Immediate freezing:** The eggs have to be dehydrated before they're frozen to prevent damage, but once they're frozen, they can be preserved for many years. Then, if you make the decision to become a parent by using these eggs, you'll move on to IVF.

- >> **In vitro fertilization (IVF):** This is the process of fertilizing the eggs outside the body so they become embryos and can be implanted. Importantly, because you can't guarantee the success of fertilization or embryo implantation, IVF can be an emotionally challenging process.

REMEMBER

TVOR adds an average of $8,000 to $15,000 per cycle to the financial cost of this process. The cost just for the freezer storage averages $300 to $700 per year. Egg retrieval and preservation is rarely covered by insurance, which is true for most of the fertility options listed in this chapter. Average base costs for a single IVF cycle are estimated to be between $14,000 and $20,000.

For trans women, trans femme people, or non-binary folks who were designated male at birth, the process of preserving genetic material is sperm freezing, or *cryopreservation*. You will be screened for any sexually transmitted infections before the sperm retrieval appointment. Then you typically masturbate into a specimen cup, and the sperm is analyzed for viability according to the following criteria:

- >> **Concentration:** How many sperm are in a specified amount of semen

- >> **Morphology:** How many of the sperm are not misshapen in some way

- >> **Motility:** How many of the sperm are swimming in the correct direction, forward

As long as the sperm sample is satisfactory, it will be frozen. It's a great idea to freeze as many samples as you can afford, as long as the analysis shows the samples are viable. If the analysis indicates serious issues with the samples, you may decide to head in a different direction with your family planning.

Estimates of the typical cost for the sperm collection process vary widely, ranging from $250 to $1,500 for analysis and freezing of a sample, and the annual storage fees are usually somewhere between $200 and $700. If you decide to use the sperm in the future, fertilization will occur through IVF or IUI (see the next section) with a partner who has a uterus or with a pregnancy *surrogate* (someone who carries the baby and gives birth to it in your place).

Relying on surrogates, donors, adoption, and other options

Using a surrogate is another option that some trans people and families have explored as their route to parenthood. Enlisting a surrogate is a complex and emotional process that has also been a huge gift for a lot of folks, cisgender and transgender alike. (*Cisgender* refers to people whose sex and gender align.)

A *surrogate* is someone, almost always a cisgender woman, who carries a baby to term and then relinquishes parental rights to you (and your partner(s) if that's your situation). Right now, the total cost for a surrogate is usually around $200,000.

There are two types of surrogates:

>> **Traditional:** This type of surrogate conceives using their own egg and someone else's sperm. They may or may not need IVF to get pregnant, and they will have to terminate parental rights when the baby is born.

>> **Gestational:** With a gestational surrogate, the egg comes from someone else. If the surrogate is working with a trans family, the egg may be harvested from you, but it doesn't have to be.

>> The surrogate has no genetic connection to the baby, and this process always requires IVF. The termination of parental rights is also part of the contract with a gestational surrogate.

WARNING

It's crucial to make sure that all the legal papers and agreements are in order when you're using a surrogate. This is one of the most critical elements if you choose this option. It's also important to do your research. When people's strong desire to have kids is involved, some people will take advantage.

Some great places to start trying to find a surrogate are surrogacy agencies, surrogacy attorneys, and surrogacy clinics, and also networking through people you already know and trust.

A donor, on the other hand, usually finishes their job before a pregnancy occurs. Human beings can donate sperm or eggs, so either or both types of donor can be involved as part of a pregnancy journey, depending on your needs.

Many families of trans men have used sperm donors to conceive, as have many lesbian couples over the decades. Any partner who has a viable uterus and ovaries can be the person to get pregnant from the donor sperm.

With an egg donor, you'll likely be using a surrogate. But with sperm you've purchased from a sperm bank, or received from a known donor, you have a few options. Some folks want to go through the process with someone they already know, and maybe even care about.

You may ask a friend or family member to be your sperm donor. If you go this route, it's important to have a clearly worded legal contract outlining the roles and responsibilities of each person.

REMEMBER

Some families want a sperm donor to be involved and part of the child's life. Others may want the relationship known to the child, but have firm boundaries that underscore that the donor isn't a parent or parental figure. The crucial thing is that everyone be in agreement, from the start, about how the family will look and the roles folks will inhabit.

A *sperm bank* (a clinic where sperm is collected, stored, and used to help people get pregnant) is a great option. If you want to avoid some of these questions. Sperm banks clearly label donors as either anonymous or willing to be known.

Throughout the selection process, you're aware of whether any future relationship with the donor is possible for your child. If this seems like a critical factor for you, you'll want to weigh the donor's willingness to be known as a more important factor than some others.

Within the last 20 or so years, as the internet has become an everyday presence in most people's lives and big online DNA databanks like Ancestry.com and 23andMe have gained popularity, some real surprises have emerged in the sperm donor landscape.

What previously seemed impossible, like locating and meeting other kids conceived with sperm from your donor, is pretty common these days.

WARNING

Uncovering the identity of an anonymous donor is also a consequence of these DNA registries. This was impossible to foresee before the introduction of at-home DNA testing. Remember that there will almost certainly be other turns in the road for some of these parenting options in the future.

If you decide to go with donor sperm, depending on a lot of factors like age, expense, any known fertility challenges, and so on, you can either begin the insemination process at home with guidance from fertility specialists, or try to maximize each sperm sample by going the healthcare provider–assisted route.

The most common method in a clinical setting is *intrauterine insemination* (IUI), in which a very small tube called a *pipette* is used to insert the sperm directly into the uterus of whoever is going to carry the baby. IUI increases the likelihood of fertilization compared to just inserting the sperm into the vagina.

If at all possible, you want to utilize a fertility practice that has at least some experience with LGBTQ people and families. Hopefully they'll even know about trans and non-binary parents.

Adoption is the process of becoming the legally recognized parent to a child who isn't your biological child. Some folks adopt kids their partner(s) had in previous relationships. Other people adopt together as a couple or multiple adults in a relationship. Still others adopt on their own.

Adoption is another example of a family-planning decision that's unique to you (or to you and your partner or partners). Common types of adoption include

>> **Agency adoption:** These adoptions, as the name implies, are conducted through a private placement agency.

>> **Foster care adoption:** Foster parenting and adoption through the foster care system are handled directly by local government agencies.

Adopting a child you're already fostering can streamline the process and may also end up being very low cost or free.

>> **Independent adoption:** This is when you use a lawyer and work with a pregnant person one-on-one, rather than through a formal agency or organization.

The expense of agency or independent adoption can range from $20,000 to $55,000.

>> **International adoption:** This means adopting a child from another country through specialized agencies, and the cost can be as high as $70,000 in some cases.

People make their families, or find their way into parenting, in many different ways. You may become a parent by getting into a long-term relationship with someone who already has kids when you meet each other. In these situations, some people end up legally adopting their partner's children, while others have incredibly close emotionally and financially supportive relationships that aren't legally formalized.

Sometimes families are formed when someone who has a child becomes unable to care for them and another person steps in to raise the child. Again, these relationships can be formalized or not, depending on the circumstances.

There are many ways to become a crucial part of a young person's life. If you feel a strong desire to do this, just remember that many roads can lead you to your destination.

Choosing to be child-free is another family-planning decision, and it's a great one. Tons of folks say that they're glad they made the choice to skip having kids, and that all the things they were able to do with their lives were totally fulfilling.

Although society has certain expectations about being in a monogamous long-term relationship, giving birth, and raising kids, those are not the only ways to have an exciting, fulfilling, and meaningful life. You only get to go around once, so hopefully you're in a position to parent, or not parent, as a conscious choice!

TIP

Family Equality (https://familyequality.org/) is an incredible organization whose website has a treasure trove of information about family planning. Check it out if this is something you are weighing right now.

Understanding How Transition Care Can Impact Your Fertility

There's some debate, and not a lot of agreement, about how transition care affects fertility. If you've already been through your natal puberty, meaning you didn't have access to puberty-blocking medications, *and* you haven't started any transition-related medical care, then any fertility issues you have are unrelated to being transgender or non-binary. This is considered the ideal time to attempt cryopreservation of sperm or eggs, because you won't have undergone any physical changes that may affect your reproductive system at this point.

REMEMBER

Parents of trans and non-binary kids are often very concerned about fertility and transition-related medical care. While some of these young people won't necessarily have an investment in genetic reproduction, it's important to explore fertility preservation options before beginning transition-related medical treatments.

So, the big question is, what changes occur after you start taking hormones? For folks who were designated female at birth, this boils down to whether the use of testosterone affects eggs in any meaningful way.

Although this question has been considered somewhat controversial, a small study from Boston IVF is often cited as proof that the issue may be overblown.

An essay by Trystan Reese sums up the findings of the study in an easy-to-read essay on the Family Equality website (https://familyequality.org/resources/testosterone-egg-health/). Here are the details of the study:

>> Twenty-six transgender men were studied.

>> They were linked to cisgender women patients with similar characteristics.

>> The trans men had to go through at least one egg harvesting cycle at one of the Boston IVF facilities.

>> No differences in egg quality and quantity between the transgender men and cisgender women were found.

>> The trans men who got pregnant had the same pregnancy experiences and outcomes as the cis women in the study.

WARNING

Testosterone is *teratogenic* (something that can cause birth defects for a fertilized egg or a fetus). While some folks believe that taking testosterone keeps you from getting pregnant, many variables can actually create the circumstances that allow someone to get pregnant while taking T. But if you want to have a baby, planned or unplanned, stop taking T as soon as possible — and definitely as soon as you know you're pregnant.

As of right now, it's also unclear whether estrogen has any effect on sperm quality or production. A known consequence of feminizing hormone therapy is decreased testicular volume and production, but the question is whether this is permanent.

Some data points to the idea that stopping your hormone therapy for three to six months allows sperm production to return to its previous level, but for some individuals this hasn't been the case. This means that most people who want to take estrogen and testosterone blockers are advised to both freeze sperm before starting down that medical route *and* still act as if they're able to get someone pregnant sexually after going on hormones. This may not sound like it makes sense, but it's definitely a better-safe-than-sorry approach.

REMEMBER

It's important to repeat that all the experts agree that you can get pregnant, or get someone pregnant, depending on your reproductive anatomy, even if you're taking hormones.

If you were born with ovaries or testes and have had them removed, then this isn't true for you. But if you still have these organs, and you have the type of sex that can result in pregnancy, it's necessary to take the appropriate precautions outlined in the next section.

Choosing a Method of Contraception That's Right for You

You may not want to take hormones or have surgery. Or maybe you'd love to have top surgery but not bottom surgery. You may be on hormone therapy, but you know there's at least some possibility of pregnancy resulting from sex. For whatever reason, you may be interested in *contraception* (various methods for preventing pregnancy).

If you were designated male at birth, contraception usually means using condoms. Folks who were designated female at birth have an array of contraceptive options. The Reproductive Health Access Project has put together an amazing table of different birth control methods (https://tinyurl.com/3s69hyxj).

If you don't ever want to get pregnant, or get someone pregnant, you can undergo surgery to ensure that outcome (for example, a vasectomy, tubal ligation, hysterectomy, and so on).

You have a lot of nonpermanent options, too. And no birth control methods are off-limits for people on testosterone — both progesterone-based and estradiol and progesterone combinations are fair game. Options include

>> **Implant:** Placed under the skin, an implant slowly releases hormones into the body over months before needing to be replaced.

>> **Intrauterine device (IUD):** There are different types, but these devices are placed directly in the uterus. They can be left in place for between 3 and 12 years, depending on which kind of IUD you use.

>> **Pill:** A daily hormonal pill to control conception is perhaps the most widely known type of birth control.

>> **Ring:** This is a flexible plastic ring that's inserted into the vagina and changed every month.

TIP

Some trans masculine and non-binary people have used contraceptive options to stop their periods, either before starting T, or if they aren't planning to use fully masculinizing hormones.

The final, sometimes difficult, aspect of family planning is pregnancy termination. Trans people who can get pregnant sometimes have to access abortion treatment as part of their family planning.

Unplanned pregnancies can happen, even on testosterone, so this is a situation that some trans folks will find themselves in if they are not ready for a baby at that time. This can be fraught, depending on where you live.

But it's further complicated for trans and non-binary people by the highly gendered framework that still often surrounds reproductive care. Chapter 7 provides some tips on finding a supportive medical provider that you can use in this case as well.

If you have options of where to go, you can research the medical providers or clinics before you visit, even calling to find out if they have seen trans patients before and how they handle things like using your chosen name.

The topics covered in this chapter involve some big decisions, but lots of other queer and trans people have walked this path before you. Whether you know that raising kids isn't for you, or you can't wait to start your parenting journey, you can find more resources out there than ever before to help you chart your way.

4

Finding Support for Your Journey

Seek support networks for your transition journey.

Access mental health resources to guide and empower you.

Chapter 12

Reaching Out for Transition Support

In this chapter we shine a spotlight on a lot of different paths you can take to find support during your transition. Hopefully you have a support system in place, including family and friends who love you and accept you. Some folks have a few trusted people in their lives who go through their transition alongside them and can smoothly make the shift with them as their gender and gender expression finally come to the surface.

But we know that isn't the reality for some of you. It's tough when folks who've cared for you all your life decide to reject you because you came out to them as transgender or non-binary. If you don't have old relationships to lean on, you can make new connections, definitely online, and ideally in your local community, too.

Your healthcare providers can also be a vital source of support during your transition, so this chapter includes some guidance on how to look for medical providers. Online directories can help you find local healthcare providers, and if you can't find anyone in your area who fits your needs, you can turn to an online provider. If you're looking for a behavioral health clinician, flip to Chapter 13.

REMEMBER

The internet has been an incredible tool for trans and non-binary people of all ages. Folks like you have used it to make new friends, fall in love, find a doctor or therapist, connect with a support group, and locate resources they need to get through their transition.

If you don't have a computer or a reliable internet connection, you may be able to use one at your local library, or possibly at a community center near you. If you have a smartphone, you can take advantage of free internet connections in public places near you. Reaching out to others locally or online can be a big step that feels intimidating, and it can also connect you to crucial people and resources you need.

Using Resources Offered by Community Organizations

Right off the bat, we suggest checking to see if any trans organizations, support groups, mutual aid groups, or advocacy groups offer services near you. These can be a great route to finding the resources you need, forging new relationships, and getting involved in community advocacy, if you're interested in that.

Our organization, the Transgender Resource Center of New Mexico (TGRCNM), which was founded in 2007, provides a huge array of resources for trans and non-binary people throughout New Mexico.

For example, TGRCNM helps folks with legal name changes, ID document updates, emergency financial assistance, support groups, nonmedical case navigation (connecting people to resources and helping them navigate systems), counseling, trans-specific items (like binders, packers, tucking supplies, and so on), and an online healthcare provider directory, among other things.

We also host trainings and social events all over New Mexico, and operate a community drop-in center in Albuquerque. All the direct services are offered free of charge, and people seeking assistance don't have to provide proof of income. You can find out more about TGRCNM online at https://tgrcnm.org/.

TGRCNM is just one transgender organization in the United States that exists to help trans folks. Gender Justice League in the state of Washington is another. GJL offers assistance with temporary stays in hotels/vacation rentals; direct financial assistance; case navigation; safety planning; and personal and policy advocacy. They plan Trans Pride Seattle, too (more info at https://www.genderjustice league.org/).

If you don't have an organization of this scope and size in your area, you can almost always find incredible community resources to connect to. To start, just Google your location along with "transgender" or "transgender resources." Another search option that works if you've updated your location settings in your web browser is "transgender resources near me."

So, for example, you can type "Cleveland transgender resources" in your browser and immediately get results for the following organizations:

>> Case Western Reserve University's LGBT Center (https://case.edu/lgbt/resources/transgender-resources)

>> Cleveland Clinic's Transgender Health and Gender Affirming Medical Services (https://tinyurl.com/yzwhmd3d)

>> The LGBT Community Center of Greater Cleveland (https://lgbtcleveland.org/programs/trans-plus/)

>> TransOhio's Support Groups page (https://www.transohio.org/supportgroups)

TIP

If searching by your city name doesn't work, try your state. You may find nearby organizations that can offer assistance, or even events or groups worth making a short trip to check out.

Some national organizations may also offer support options and resources that appeal to you. At the time of writing, an online search for "national transgender resources" returned the following results:

>> Advocates for Trans Equality, or A4TE (https://transequality.org/)

>> GLAAD (https://glaad.org/transgender/resources/)

>> PFLAG (https://pflag.org/resource/transgender-resources/)

>> The Trevor Project (https://www.thetrevorproject.org/)

>> Trans Lifeline (https://translifeline.org/hotline/)

>> Transgender Law Center (https://transgenderlawcenter.org/)

>> World Professional Association for Transgender Health, or WPATH (https://www.wpath.org/resources/general)

TIP

Trans Resources (`https://trans-resources.info/`) is an amazing website that offers a directory with links to advocacy organizations, support groups, and legal resources across the world. You can search by country or state to find resources near you. The site is continuously being updated as more resources for trans and non-binary people are identified.

Finding a Supportive Healthcare Provider

REMEMBER

For the last 50 years or so, the most reliable way to find a trans-friendly healthcare provider has been word of mouth from other trans and non-binary people. You may get recommendations face to face, in support groups, or from local trans organizations or advocacy workers. Check with several different sources if you have to. (See Chapter 7 for more info about healthcare for transgender and non-binary patients.)

You can also use the internet to find compassionate healthcare providers to support your gender-transition journey. For example, our organization, TGRCNM, has an online provider directory that's specific to New Mexico.

Be sure to check whether you have a local community center or other local resources that can offer some hard-earned knowledge about which providers are safe and accessible. Some of the bigger online provider directories are

>> GLMA's LGBTQ+ Healthcare Directory (`https://www.glma.org/find_a_provider.php`)

>> OutCare Health (`https://www.outcarehealth.org/`)

>> Trans in the South (`https://southernequality.org/resources/transinthesouth/`)

>> WPATH's Provider Directory (`https://www.wpath.org/provider/search`)

What if you don't have any nearby healthcare providers to work with? Whether you live in a rural area or don't have reliable transportation or face some other barrier, you may have difficulty getting to in-person appointments with a trans-friendly provider. Luckily, you now have some good online healthcare options, including

>> Circle Medical (`https://tinyurl.com/57pzs65k`)

>> FOLX (`https://www.folxhealth.com/`)

>> Plume (`https://getplume.co/`)

These online healthcare providers have been lifesaving resources for a whole lot of folks who have many reasons for not being able to see a medical provider in person.

Expanding Your Personal Connections

It's a great idea to surround yourself with folks who accept and affirm you as you are. If you don't currently have anyone in your life you can relate to or connect with, check out our suggestions in the following sections.

Turning to your friends and family

You may already have folks in your life who love you a lot and can't wait to support you as you transition. If you're lucky enough to have a handful of trusted people around you — whether they're people you're biologically related to, other close family and friends you grew up with, or great friends you met later in life — make sure you reach out to them during this time.

If you decide to undergo hormone therapy, you're going to go through puberty again. The various parts of the transition process go so much better when you have supportive people to talk to. Your existing relationships can be some of your best assets.

For some folks, though, deciding to move forward with gender transition means that many of the people in their life may not be around anymore. Family and friends who have been important to you may turn away, leaving gaps in your support system, or you may just be interested in making new connections with trans, non-binary, or cisgender folks who are comfortable with you and your gender path. (*Cisgender* refers to people whose sex and gender match.)

You can use some of the same strategies we suggest earlier in this chapter to find transgender and non-binary support groups in your area or online. Some websites with online support groups include

>> The Trevor Project (https://www.thetrevorproject.org/) - youth

>> Plume (https://getplume.co/support-groups/)

>> Trans Advocacy & Care Team (https://www.yourtact.org/)

You can also look for new friends in places other than support groups. A lot of transgender and non-binary folks face challenges with anxiety, but putting yourself out there can be a risk worth taking. You can start slowly and even do some of your engagement with others online if that's more comfortable.

Some ideas for making new connections include

» **Search online for a social group to join.** Meetup (https://www.meetup.com/lp/friendship-and-socializing/) provides links to social groups for people that are interested in hiking, dancing, eating out, knitting, joining a kickball team, reading, playing Dungeons & Dragons, and so much more.

Many of the social gatherings are designated as LGBTQ get-togethers, but you don't have to go to a specifically LGBTQ meetup. The website also has listings for online events and groups where you don't have to show up in person.

» **Check out other online communities.** Some transgender and non-binary people have found communities on general social media apps like Instagram.

Seeking out folks on these apps who have shared interests with you can be a place to start.

» **Volunteer.** Doing something that helps others can make you feel incredible and may be a great way to meet folks who are interested in the same things you are. As a trans or non-binary person, you need to exercise good judgment about the local volunteer opportunities that feel safe to you.

But donating some of your time to causes like animal shelters, environmental welfare, voting rights and political campaigns, early childhood education, and LGBTQ issues can help you get your momentum going.

» **Take a class.** You may be interested in a ukulele class at a local community center or vocational classes at the community college. You can audit classes at a nearby university, or even online.

Taking classes in subjects that interest you can broaden your horizons and lead you to like-minded folks. Even in online classes, students are often put into smaller groups for discussions or team projects, giving you the opportunity to get to know your classmates better.

» **Join a gym.** Exercise isn't for everyone, but if you're looking to get in shape, try a gym! If you can't afford a gym, check out the local community center or YMCA for an inexpensive, but communal, place to work out. Once you start going, make an effort to talk to others.

» **Put down your devices.** It's difficult in the modern world, but if you don't default to staring at your screen when you're on public transportation, waiting in line, at the medical clinic, walking your dog, or going about your everyday business, you have a much greater chance of sparking up a conversation with someone you may find interesting.

Researchers have found that loneliness has similar health risks as cigarette smoking. Nobody is to blame for their own loneliness when social isolation is so clearly a structural defect in modern culture. But doing all you can to try to make connections with other people benefits your physical and mental health as well as your social life.

Getting involved with faith-based practices and communities

For many LGBTQ people, religious and faith traditions are a source of profound abuse and wounding. Some people in the transgender and non-binary communities cannot imagine finding solace, or even being safe approaching, a church, synagogue, mosque, or *sangha* (a Buddhist community). But for others, these traditions are deep cultural and family identifiers, and can be a well of resilience, compassion, and self-love in their life.

Transgender and non-binary Christians may find themselves in a bind in terms of locating an affirming, loving community to join. Gaychurch.org (https://www.gaychurch.org/) is a terrific website that has a directory of LGBTQ-affirming churches, broken down by state and searchable by location. The site has a lot of other excellent resources for trans or non-binary Christians trying to figure out where to plug in.

Once you locate a church (or churches) in your area on the gaychurch.org directory (or by word of mouth or some other way), you can check their website and even reach out to the pastor with a brief email.

Some churches with LGBTQ-welcoming congregations are still behind the curve on trans inclusion and acceptance, so don't be afraid to ask before you go. Better to get an awkward or defensive email from the pastor than to show up at a church that really isn't ready for you.

Each Christian denomination uses different language, like affirming, to signal LGBTQ acceptance; becoming familiar with these terms can help you in your search. Wikipedia has published a series on Christianity and LGBTQ issues that includes an article with an extensive list of affirming and welcoming churches (https://tinyurl.com/38whhxkz).

Transgender and non-binary people who are Jewish may also be deeply involved and invested in their faith, not at all interested in practicing Judaism, or somewhere in the middle. Keshet (https://tinyurl.com/2w2hyfn4), which has an online directory of affirming synagogues, rabbis, and other resources that are inclusive, is a great place to start if you're looking for a temple, or just a Jewish community that's safe and accessible.

Although Islam is often viewed as intolerant of LGBTQ people, as with any other enormous group of people, Muslims around the world have varying opinions. Finding an open and accepting mosque can be a challenge, but Muslims for Progressive Values (https://www.mpvusa.org/) has a lot of great resources on their website that may help you start connecting with others of your faith and building a community.

Buddhism, likewise, can be mixed in terms of acceptance and inclusion for LGBTQ folks, but many sanghas will be happy to have you even if they're not explicitly affirming. Here are some good online resources and practices to check out:

>> Rainbodhi (https://rainbodhi.org/)

>> Rainbow Sangha (https://tinyurl.com/54azs9nr)

>> Undefended Dharma (https://marystancavage.org/)

>> Tricycle (https://tricycle.org/category/lgbtq/)

TIP

The Human Rights Campaign has a web page that lists the resources covered in this section, plus quite a few more (https://www.hrc.org/resources/faith-resources).

You can try to reach out in many different ways to receive the support you need and deserve during this time of intense change in your life. We hope this chapter gives you some starting points.

IN THIS CHAPTER

» Locating mental health
  care providers

» Exploring different types of support

» Reaching out to suicide
  prevention resources

Chapter **13**

Obtaining Mental Health Support

Transgender and non-binary people currently report much higher levels of all kinds of medical and mental health challenges than *cisgender* folks (whose gender and sex align). This higher risk to your mental health is not *because* you're trans or non-binary; it's a natural response to having a minority characteristic that's still subjected to stigma, discrimination, and violence.

In this chapter, we explore the world of therapy and behavioral health. We start with the basics — finding a mental health care provider — and then cover some other behavioral health resources that may be helpful to you. And because trans and non-binary people have a higher risk of suicide and suicidal thoughts, we highlight some resources you can seek out if you're considering self-harm.

Seeking Out Mental Health Care

Trying to figure out when you need help with your mental health, and how to get it, can be overwhelming! A lot of people are discouraged from talking about their problems, or even their feelings. It's easy to make the case that there's still a significant amount of stigma attached to mental health issues and challenges in the

United States. Even as a greater array of resources becomes available, it can feel intimidating to reach out for help.

How do you know when you need help?

Most parents aren't taught how to develop emotional bonds with their children, and there's a lack of infrastructure to support good parenting skills. This means that a lot of kids don't get what they need emotionally as they're growing up, even if they have a good childhood and all their material needs are met. Trans and non-binary people have an additional layer of disconnection that comes from being different in a way that still isn't completely understood and accepted.

Lack of emotional security from caregivers in childhood can be correlated with depression, anxiety, and other mental health challenges. So, even if you're managing to get by in your life and fulfilling your daily responsibilities, you may be carrying around a mental health burden you don't have to carry. Looking into any of the approaches listed in this chapter may open the door to a different experience of yourself and others and more emotional freedom.

In other words, it's really never a bad idea (for most people, but especially for trans and non-binary folks) to have a safe, trusted professional you can talk to and work things out with. Even if you don't particularly feel bad, it can be emotionally freeing to have the support of a good therapist or counselor. Some specific signs that it's time to reach out for help include

>> **Overwhelming emotions:** Feelings are normal, and huge life events like gender transition can engender *lots* of different emotions in you. But if you feel like your feelings are too much to handle, a supportive therapist can be a big help.

>> **Coping mechanisms that are hurting you or others:** Everyone has different ways they cope with stressful situations, but if your coping strategies are hurting your relationships, daily tasks, work, or school, that can point to a need for some outside help.

>> **Your loved ones are worried:** It can be hard to have folks you love tell you that you're struggling. It can seem like a criticism or bring up feelings of shame. But these are the people who love you and they are the best mirrors for knowing when it's time.

>> **Difficulty maintaining your normal life:** This is different from just needing a break from things. If you find that you are consistently struggling to do the things you usually like to do, or need to do, reaching out is a great idea.

If you do feel you're in crisis, then it's definitely time to reach out. Getting into therapy, or engaging with other behavioral health strategies is great, but also check out the crisis lines listed later in the chapter (see "Turning to Suicide Prevention Resources").

Finding a therapist or mental health care provider

Honestly, it's so much better to get into a great relationship with a therapist when you *aren't* in crisis. But if you don't already have a mental health care provider, you can start your search by talking with trans, non-binary, or other LGBTQ folks you know. They're very likely to have already done the research to find out if a provider is friendly and knowledgeable about trans issues and people.

If you have a local transgender or LGBTQ resource center or community center, or a group like PFLAG or a state equality organization, these can also be first stops for a referral. They may even have a counselor on staff, as we do at Transgender Resource Center of New Mexico.

If the mental health resources are limited in your area, the provider themself may be the biggest factor in your decision. However, if you have more options on providers to try, you'll want to narrow down your criteria to help with your search.

Here are some important considerations before you begin looking:

>> **Experience:** Does the provider have a lot of experience with trans and non-binary people? Maybe they have just a little experience with trans issues, but they're enthusiastic and accessible.

There's no right answer, but you need to know what you're looking for, ideally.

>> **Insurance:** Whether you have insurance, the type of insurance you have, and what your plan covers are all details that will impact your choice.

>> **Location:** Your transportation options and how far away the provider is can be significant factors in your decision.

>> **Therapeutic approach:** If you haven't experienced therapy before, it's easy to imagine that all therapists do some version of the same thing. That's not true, though. Therapeutic approaches and types of treatment are varied, and you need to find the different components of your best mental health regimen.

We provide a link to more information on various types of therapy in the later section "Types of counseling."

You'll probably have lots of questions for a potential new mental health care provider, and it's a great idea to make a list of those concerns. Some therapists offer a free first visit or consultation so that you can both evaluate whether the relationship seems like a good fit. You can take that opportunity to ask all of your questions before making a final decision.

How do you find a mental health care provider other than asking folks? We recommend searching through the following directories:

>> WPATH Provider Directory (https://www.wpath.org/provider/search)

>> Psychology Today, which includes transgender as a filter on its search tool (https://www.psychologytoday.com/)

>> National Queer & Trans Therapists of Color Network (https://nqttcn.com/en/)

TIP

If there aren't a lot of great therapists in your area, don't feel you have to settle for someone you don't click with. Trust your gut! If the therapist doesn't seem to care about you or appears more interested in billing you for their time than helping you, you don't have to go back.

If you feel like you're going to have to educate them about transgender or non-binary issues, they may not be the best therapist for you. Instead, you can check out online counseling platforms such as LGBTQ Therapy Space, the Trans+ Therapy Library, FOLX, and Plume Health. Good mental health services are out there, even if you have to access them online.

Types of counseling

All mental health therapy isn't the same; there are a lot of different therapeutic approaches and modalities. You may not know exactly which is best for you going into the process, but it's a good idea to have some familiarity with the most common types of counseling as you try to find your provider.

Psychology Today offers a pretty thorough guide to the different therapeutic approaches at https://www.psychologytoday.com/us/types-of-therapy. Some examples are

>> Somatic therapy

>> Eye Movement Desensitization and Reprocessing (EMDR)

>> Internal Systems therapy

>> Transpersonal therapy

LOWERING YOUR RISK OF MENTAL HEALTH ISSUES

Even if you haven't been the victim of physical violence, and even if you have a loving, supportive family, being trans in the United States still takes a toll on you. A review on the health website Medical News Today references several studies that show significant increases in depression, anxiety, stress, substance misuse, and suicide for transgender folks compared to cisgender people.

Another critical thing to remember is that these mental health inequities are compounded by any additional vulnerable traits you have — in other words, other characteristics that expose you to discrimination or violence.

For example, race and gender are major indicators that you may experience discrimination, but this also tracks along the lines of disability, nationality, neurodivergence, and body type and size, among other traits.

The data, as well as many people's lived experiences, makes it clear that trans women and trans feminine people have much worse outcomes. For example, Black trans women reported twice the rate of ever being fired for being trans – 26% – than the overall respondent group – 13% – in the 2015 U.S. Trans Survey than trans men and trans masculine people. And Black and Indigenous trans folks consistently experience much worse treatment than white trans people.

But it's important to remember that none of these traits *cause* discrimination or violence. Rather, this type of mistreatment is the product of a dominant culture that still struggles with racism and sexism.

You have lots of treatment choices and strategies to lower your risk of mental health issues due to the societal challenges you face. It's important to reach out for help in dealing with any difficulties you encounter, because your mental health directly affects your physical health. Make sure you have the tools you need to maintain a healthy mind and body!

Experimenting with Other Behavioral Health Resources

You can try other strategies for strengthening your mental and emotional health beyond traditional talk therapy. The options in the following list can be a great supplement to traditional therapy, or even an alternate therapeutic treatment.

Many of them have been shown to have real benefits for people who utilize them, but others haven't been studied as well yet.

>> **Acupuncture:** Many folks swear by acupuncture, a treatment involving the insertion of needles into certain areas of the body. Originating in Asia, it has a long history of being beneficial for human health, and may also help with stress, anxiety, and emotional regulation.

>> **Animal therapy:** Animal therapies, including therapeutic work with horses, have a great body of evidence to back them up. Connecting with animals can ease the pent-up fear and anxiety you may have from past mistreatment.

Animals may also be a source of comfort outside the therapeutic setting. Adopting a pet, or even volunteering with a local animal shelter, can help you get outside yourself, and bask in the unconditional love that pets often provide.

>> **Art therapy:** You can find some great art therapists to work with, and many conventional therapists incorporate art and other creative activities into the counseling they offer. Or just creating art on your own or with friends can be incredibly therapeutic.

Many artists have talked about how creating art saved their life and gave them an outlet for their repressed feelings about traumatic experiences. You don't have to have any special talent to enjoy creating art and to benefit from the creative process.

>> **EMDR:** *Eye movement desensitization and reprocessing (EMDR)* therapy utilizes bilateral stimulation to help the brain reprocess traumatic memories and experiences. *Bilateral stimulation* just means stimulating both sides of the brain in short intervals, but not simultaneously.

This can be done with lights to trigger movement of the eyes, or with buzzing paddles held in each hand. EMDR is performed by a licensed therapist, so use the tips in the previous section to find someone who does it.

>> **Massage:** Therapeutic touch can be a profound addition to your wellness regimen. Many people don't get enough human touch, and that may be especially true for trans and non-binary people.

Again, be sure that you work with a massage therapist who has experience with, and is welcoming to, trans people. And don't worry about having to take off all your clothes. Any good massage therapist will want you to wear whatever you need to in order to be comfortable.

>> **Meditation:** Meditation has been used for hundreds of years to help heal the mind and rewire the neural pathways. Don't be intimated — you can find lots of apps and websites to guide you through the process. Meditating for just five minutes a day has been shown to have a big impact on mental health.

TIP

There are many types of meditation, but the most common in the U.S. is called *insight meditation*. Contrary to popular belief, this doesn't involve clearing or emptying your mind. It's just the practice of trying to focus on your breath (or another type of anchor if the breath work makes you anxious) while knowing that your mind will get distracted. You continue to gently bring your mind back to your breath, even counting your breaths in and out, and calling your mind back when it runs off (the way you would a young puppy).

>> **Music therapy:** Learning to play an instrument can put your brain to work and give you something to focus on other than your gender or your transition. If you're lucky enough to be able to make music with other people, you'll get the benefits of human connection and music therapy at the same time.

Listening to music, even alone in your room, can give you the feeling of being connected to other people who relate to what you're going through. Some great trans artists are currently making music, but you don't have to limit yourself to their work — listen to the music you love!

>> **Neurofeedback:** This exists under the umbrella of biofeedback, and has worked really well for some people. It is also called EEG (electroencephalo-gram) biofeedback because you are fitted with the same types of electrodes used in an EEG.

The provider watches your brainwaves on a screen and the computer program guides your brain activity to its optimal state. *Psychology Today* has a pretty balanced article describing the pros and cons of neurofeedback (https://www.psychologytoday.com/us/therapy-types/neurofeedback).

>> **Psychedelic therapy:** The medical evidence to support this treatment isn't in yet, so approach psychedelic therapy with caution. However, many folks have reported significant mental and emotional benefits from safe usage of different types of psychedelic medications, such as MDMA, psyilcybin, and ketamine.

An article in the *Journal of the American Medical Association* gives a good overview of psychedelic therapy. Even though this is based on a single small study, the authors report that these therapies are promising (https://jamanetwork.com/journals/jama/fullarticle/2808951).

You may also want to look into microdosing, which is using small amounts of psilocybin, for example, to avoid the strong psychedelic experience while experiencing some therapeutic benefits.

>> **Support groups:** Although some support groups are led by licensed thera-pists, a lot of them are *peer-facilitated*, which just means folks like you lead and help organize the group. You can find in-person and online support groups for all kinds of transgender and non-binary people, as well as families and loved ones.

But don't limit yourself to trans groups. Many different types of support groups can be a good fit for your interests or circumstances. You'll have to make sure that these groups feel welcoming to you as a trans person, but they can be a great place to make friends and form connections with people who have shared life experiences or interests.

>> **Yoga:** More research is needed, but some promising studies back up the idea that yoga is an effective treatment for mental health issues.

And more importantly, people throughout history have anecdotally reported significant mental health benefits from practicing yoga's physical postures and breathing techniques.

We could add a lot more to this list, including spending time in nature, making social connections with other people, eating a healthy diet, exercising, getting plenty of sleep, practicing mindful gratitude, and so on. The bottom line is, if something really boosts your mental health, put it on your list of helpful strategies!

TIP

If an alternative mental health treatment or practice sounds appealing to you, give it a try. Be patient — even if it doesn't yield the results you're hoping for, it may lead you closer to your goals or simply ease your mind. One member of our team has gotten terrific results from EMDR, while another has engaged with it consistently without seeing the same benefits. No one thing will work for everyone, but something out there will probably be of benefit to your brain and body.

Turning to Suicide Prevention Resources

Unfortunately, the data shows that trans and non-binary people are at an exponentially higher risk for suicidal thoughts and behavior than the general population. The percentages vary based on the dataset, but the risk of suicide for trans folks is consistently two to four times higher. Remember, this is *not* because the suicidal person is transgender or non-binary; it's a product of the stigma, discrimination, and violence faced by trans and non-binary people in almost every setting of public and private life.

TIP

A really great, usually 45-minute training called QPR, which stands for *question, persuade, refer*, is offered all over the country by trained instructors, usually free of charge. Much like CPR, it's training that allows regular people to step in and try to help if someone expresses suicidal thoughts. You can search online for "QPR near me" to find opportunities to take this training. This type of grassroots preparation can save a lot of lives.

If *you* are feeling suicidal, now or in the future, please reach out. It can be extremely hard to take any step in that moment to get help, but the people you're close to will be forever grateful that you did. Feeling that nobody loves you or cares about you is almost certainly just the product of the emotions you're experiencing.

There are folks out there who care if you live or die, and all your future friends and loved ones are hanging in the balance, too. Don't let shame or fear get in the way of putting your hand out for help at this critical moment.

REMEMBER

When folks who have made a suicide attempt and survive are interviewed afterward, they almost never express regret about their survival. They're often bewildered by the fact that they got so close to the irrevocable step of death. Give yourself that chance.

Some places you can reach out to (some are available 24 hours a day) include the following hotlines and crisis intervention services:

>> Trans Lifeline (https://translifeline.org/ or 877-565-8860)

>> LGBT National Help Center (https://lgbthotline.org/national-hotline/ or 888-843-4564)

>> Crisis Text Line, which is not LGBT-specific (https://www.crisistextline.org/text-us/ or text 741741)

>> BlackLine, a crisis hotline that will help anyone but is geared toward people of color and the Black LGBTQ community (https://www.callblackline.com/ or 800-604-5841)

>> National Suicide Crisis Lifeline (https://988lifeline.org/ or call or text 988)

You can also get in touch with a *warmline*, which isn't specifically a crisis intervention service, but is still a place to reach out to for help. Some warmlines you can contact to talk to someone are

>> Trans Advice (https://transadvice.org/)

>> The Trevor Project (thetrevorproject.org or 866-488-7386)

>> THRIVE Lifeline (https://thrivelifeline.org/)

REMEMBER

Even for cisgender people, the dominant culture doesn't always cultivate and nurture human connection and well-being. But in the darkest moments, there's always the possibility for something different, something better. Please reach out, explore the resources in this book, or offer your hand to someone else who may need it.

This isn't easy stuff, but you can get through the dark times, and change your life. You may not be able to imagine a brighter future today, but it could be out there.

5

The Part of Tens

IN THIS PART . . .

Discover influential transgender and non-binary figures throughout history.

Explore key topics to address with your healthcare provider.

Locate trans-friendly organizations.

Find impactful ways to support transgender and non-binary people.

Chapter **14**

Ten (or So) Famous Transgender and Non-Binary People

Transgender and non-binary people have always existed, and you are part of a long, unbroken thread of special people throughout human history. In this chapter, we introduce you to some really amazing transgender and non-binary people. They come from different eras and are known for different things. We hope they inspire you!

REMEMBER

Even in places and times where others have tried to suppress or get rid of them, trans people have survived.

Leslie Feinberg

Les Feinberg, born in 1949, was most famously the author of the pivotal novel *Stone Butch Blues*. Feinberg used zie/hir pronouns, so that's how zie is referred to here.

Feinberg was, in hir own words, "an anti-racist white, working-class, secular Jewish, transgender, lesbian, female, revolutionary communist." Zie was a long-time activist and author who had an outsize impact on many trans and non-binary people, including at least one member of our writing team. Zie died at home in Syracuse, New York, on November 15, 2014, with hir partner and spouse of 22 years, Minnie Bruce Pratt, at hir side.

Compton's Cafeteria "Rioters"

In August 1966, a group of transgender women and drag queens, many of whom were surviving through street-based sex work, got together to hang out and get off the street for a bit at a place called Compton's Cafeteria in San Francisco's Tenderloin district. They had been subjected to police harassment and violence, and the cafeteria was taking discriminatory action to try to prevent them from being in the establishment. This resulted in one of the first LGBTQ riots in the 1960s.

These riots, including the 1969 Stonewall riots in New York City, sparked a lot of political advocacy and action in the years following. You can find out more about the Compton's Cafeteria riot in the documentary *Screaming Queens: The Riot at Compton's Cafeteria*, and on the GLBT Historical Society's website (https://www.glbthistory.org/newsletter-blog-2020/08-feature).

We'wha

We'wha was a member of the Zuni Pueblo who was referred to by the Zuni term lhamana, which described people who were designated male at birth but who took on social and cultural roles usually occupied by women. Lhamana often wear a mix of men's and women's clothing. We'wha was very respected as a spiritual leader and served as a cultural ambassador from Zuni to Washington, D.C. in the late 1800s. We'wha lived from 1849 to 1896.

Brian Michael Smith

Brian Michael Smith is an accomplished Black transgender actor and advocate for LGBTQ people. He is famous for playing Toine Wilkins on *Queen Sugar*, a show produced by Ava DuVernay, as well as firefighter Paul Strickland on *9-1-1: Lone Star*, created by Ryan Murphy and Brad Falchuk. He gives one of his sweetest performances in the short film *Tell-by Date* (https://www.tellbydate.com/). You can find him on all the major social media platforms and IMDB.

Sarah McBride

Sarah McBride, a longtime advocate and activist, was the first openly transgender state senator in the United States. In November 2024 she became the first out transgender person elected to the U.S. Congress when she picked up the at-large congressional seat in her home state of Delaware.

Earlier in her life, McBride was the national spokesperson for the Human Rights Campaign, and she is the author of *Tomorrow Will Be Different*, a beautiful and affecting memoir centering her love story with her late husband, Andrew Cray, also a dedicated transgender advocate. You can find out more about her at her official website (https://www.sarahmcbride.com/about).

Alok Vaid-Menon

Alok Vaid-Menon is a multi-talented writer, performer, and activist. They have a long history of advocating for trans and non-binary people, and for body and gender diversity. They were born in 1991 and raised in College Station, Texas. Some selected titles by Alok are *Beyond the Gender Binary, Femme in Public,* and *Your Wound/My Garden*. Notable performances include the Edinburgh Fringe Festival, the Kennedy Center for the Performing Arts, and headlining the Netflix Is a Joke and Just for Laughs festivals. They are the subject of the docu-short *ALOK*, executive produced by Jodie Foster and directed by Alex Hedison, which made its debut at the Sundance Film Festival in 2024. They are cited as a big influence by lots of trans and non-binary people. You can find out more about Alok at their website https://www.alokvmenon.com/.

Janelle Monáe

Janelle Monáe is a musician, actor, songwriter, performance artist, and celebrity who came out as non-binary in 2022. They are famous for rocking tuxedos and their signature black-and-white red carpet looks, as well as an android, sci-fi aesthetic. In a 2022 interview, the *Los Angeles Times* reported that "the singer identifies as nonbinary", and quoted them as saying, "My pronouns are free-ass motherfucker, and they/them, her/she."

Kim Coco Iwamoto

Kim Coco Iwamoto is a transgender politician and advocate from Hawaii. Recognized by President Barack Obama as a Champion of Change, she was elected to two terms on the Hawaii Board of Education, and was a Democratic primary candidate for lieutenant governor in 2018. In November 2024 she became the first openly transgender state legislator in Hawaii. You can check out her website at https://www.votekimcoco.com/.

Amelio Robles Ávila

Amelio Robles Ávila was born in 1889, when he was designated female at birth. However, he joined the army at age 24, and two years into his service adopted a masculine style of dress and told the people around him to treat him as a man. He was well-respected and obtained the rank of colonel. After the Mexican Revolution he married his wife, adopted a daughter, and lived to 95 years old, dying in 1984. A researcher who studied Colonel Robles reported that if folks used a feminine address toward him, he threatened them with a gun! Making Queer History (https://www.makingqueerhistory.com/) is a great source to learn more.

Lucy Hicks Anderson

Lucy Hicks Anderson was a Black transgender woman who lived in Oxnard, California, from 1920 to 1946. She was married to two different men, and ran a successful brothel in Oxnard for many years before being arrested in 1945. She was tried for and convicted of perjury after a public outing brought about by the arrest. She remains one of the earliest recorded Black trans people in the United States.

The Wachowskis

Sisters Lilly and Lana Wachowski are writers, directors, and producers who are both transgender women. They have collaborated on video games, comic books, movies, and television shows. Some of their very famous and influential works include *The Matrix* movies, *Bound*, *V for Vendetta*, *Cloud Atlas*, and the terrific series *Sense8*. Their projects often deal with trans themes and issues, even if they aren't explicitly about trans people. *Sense8*, though, has a trans actress playing a trans role, in a series that features many LGBTQ storylines.

Chapter 15

Ten Essential Topics to Discuss with Your Healthcare Provider

You may notice that a lot of this book deals with healthcare and health-related issues. Healthcare is an important part of life, especially for folks who undertake any medical transition steps. If you take hormones or have gender-affirming surgery, you need to have healthcare providers you trust. But if you've had negative experiences in the past, you know that building trust with medical providers can be tough. Chapters 7, 12, and 13 offer advice about finding, assessing, and selecting medical and behavioral health providers; in this chapter you find some recommendations and reminders about the most important things you can talk about with these folks once they begin caring for you.

REMEMBER

The right medical providers, locally or online, are going to be partners in your healthcare and advocates for what's best for you. Some of the topics covered in this chapter may help you weed out healthcare professionals who don't suit you, but most of the content is meant to prompt conversations that allow a trusted provider to support you by taking care of your health.

Communicating Your Pronouns

It seems like this goes without saying, but you have to be comfortable enough with a new healthcare provider to tell them your chosen name and pronouns, even if that information isn't reflected in your legal documentation. This is one of the topics that helps you determine if the medical provider is a good fit or not.

Although there are good medical providers out there who work in places where the staff aren't all up to speed, this can be a great indicator of the safety of a medical practice or clinic. Staff should not only have good training on trans and non-binary people and pronouns, they should also have a good working knowledge of how to be aware and inclusive of trans people on the phone.

Discussing Preventive Care

This is also a big topic covered under a short heading. Talking to your medical provider about preventive care can range from discussing any cancer risks you face and screenings you need, to conferring about *polycythemia* (overproduction of red blood cells that thickens the blood), which can occur in trans masculine folks on testosterone. Conversations about vaccinations, bone density, liver function, blood pressure, vascular health, and diabetes are important for transgender and non-binary patients and their providers to have.

REMEMBER

Even though it may feel deeply uncomfortable, the rule of thumb is, if you have a body part, you should get it screened. That means screenings for breast, prostate, and reproductive cancers, as well as sexually transmitted infection (STI) screenings. Talk to your provider about possible accommodations or support when you're having these tests done. Don't be afraid to ask to have a friend with you during an exam or screening, to request that you be allowed to keep some of your clothing on, or to ask the provider to use a pediatric *speculum* (the instrument inserted into the body during a pelvic exam) if you're someone who doesn't have a positive relationship with their vagina.

Providing Your Health History

Talking to your medical provider about your health history can make a big difference in their ability to meaningfully support you. If they don't know about silicone injections that you may have had, previous illnesses or surgeries (that may or may not be related to your trans status), or black-market hormones you've taken, then they won't be able to quickly respond if you have challenges down the road connected to those past health and health access issues. You may not be familiar with your genetic family, but if you are, talking to your healthcare team about family medical history can provide crucial information that factors into screening decisions and other choices you make with the practitioner's support.

If the provider is right for you, you'll hopefully feel like you're able to share other deeply personal information with them. This would include (but certainly isn't limited to) the following:

>> Relationship status, including having more than one sexual partner at a time (also called *polyamory*) and sexual orientation information

>> HIV status

>> Substance use

>> Mental health challenges

>> Personal life issues, such as financial problems, domestic violence, or housing struggles

>> "Embarrassing" health issues like having problems going to the bathroom, unusual odors, or frustrations with your sex life

REMEMBER

More and more these days electronic medical records (EMRs) and electronic health records are capturing what's called an *organ inventory*. This means that as part of the electronic intake, patients are universally asked which organs they have of the set of body parts that aren't common to all sexes. For instance, patients are asked if they have

>> Cervix

>> Uterus

>> Testes/testicles

>> Prostate

>> Breasts

>> Other organs or body parts that are considered sex-specific

You can give this information to your healthcare provider even if their EMR system hasn't caught up with the times yet.

Consulting about Hair Issues

Some trans and non-binary folks are deeply concerned about different aspects of their hair. Some trans feminine people are worried about pattern baldness they may have already experienced. At the same time, if you are trans feminine and didn't have access to puberty blockers, you may be worrying about how you'll get rid of your unwanted facial or body hair. Similarly, trans masculine people often inquire about how to grow facial hair more quickly, but many are also apprehensive about thinning hair and balding.

You may be tired of reading this by now, but every trans and non-binary person is different. So, if you're a trans woman or on the femme side and non-binary and you love your beard or have no self-consciousness about your balding, that's terrific. And if you're a trans man who loves your long, beautiful hair, rock that hairstyle!

TIP

More effective and affordable treatments for balding are available these days, so hair growth is definitely something to ask your medical provider about. They may also have a good referral for laser hair removal or electrolysis. These treatments are gradually being moved into the category of procedures insurance covers, so do your research on that, too.

Getting Thorough Information about Transition Care

The different healthcare providers you work with may have a hand in various aspects of your health, and some may be experts on hormones and their risks and benefits. If so, utilize their expertise! But the conversation about hormone therapy is especially important to have with your primary care provider (PCP), because in the best-case scenario they're the person who should be administering your hormones.

Of course, *you* need to be the foremost expert on the transition care you want, if you have the ability and resources to gather that information. This book is a huge first step in finding out about hormones, surgeries, and other transition-related healthcare, and Part 3 is your jumping-off point. Your PCP is your partner in all this, though, so having honest, open conversations about your transition goals, even if they change, is critical.

Navigating the Insurance Maze

You may need the help of your healthcare providers to navigate the sometimes thorny world of insurance. Although insurance coverage of gender-affirming care vacillates, in general, the carriers have gotten more inclusive of these treatments in the last ten years or so. Since 2010, when the Affordable Care Act restricted discrimination against LGBTQ people, the push to get these treatments covered really began in earnest. Now, in some states you can access hormones, surgeries, hair removal, and even voice training through your insurance plan.

Talk to your provider about whether they accept your insurance and if they're aware of any charges you may not be expecting. You also need to be able to talk to them, and receive reasonably timely responses, about helping you use your insurance to get other treatments you want. They may be called on to provide referrals or to play a part in preauthorization for those treatments.

Easing into Sexual Health Conversations

Of all the sensitive topics in this chapter, your sexual health may very well be the one you have the most difficulty discussing with someone — even a medical professional. Talking about medical issues that involve your genitals or reproductive organs, challenges with your *libido* (sex drive), family planning, and contraception is incredibly important, but these conversations can be embarrassing or make you feel vulnerable and exposed. This can be especially true if you need to undergo any kind of exam in order to get help.

TIP

Think about whether you can do anything to make talking about this topic easier for you, like writing down your questions before your visit, bringing a friend/loved one to your appointment, or practicing the conversation with someone you trust. Some key sexual health issues that trans and non-binary folks may need to discuss include

>> **Cancer screenings:** You need to be screened for cancers of the uterus, cervix, prostate, and breast if you have these parts.

>> **Effects of surgery on sexuality:** Talk to your surgeon/PCP about any impact surgery may have on your libido, the mechanics of sex, and your sexual experiences.

>> **Family planning/fertility/contraception:** Your healthcare provider should be willing to counsel you on this subject. Check out Chapter 11 for a lot of info on family planning that can prepare you for this discussion.

>> **HIV treatment and prevention:** If you're HIV positive, you need to be open and honest with your healthcare provider and make them part of your care team. If you're HIV negative, you may be interested in preventing future HIV infection. The right provider will want to help you get on *PrEP* (pre-exposure prophylaxis, or medication you take regularly to prevent HIV infection) rather than discourage you from taking it.

>> **Libido:** Hormone therapy can have intense effects on your sex drive, in all directions. This is part of puberty, but your provider can likely help if you're experiencing any problems.

>> **Pelvic pain:** These days you hear a little bit more about this type of pain, but it's still something trans masculine folks often don't talk about. If you're experiencing pelvic pain during sex or otherwise, discuss it with your medical provider.

>> **Sexual partners and sexual pleasure:** Your provider can better support you if you talk to them about your sexual partners (that is, the number and types of people you have sex with). Although it's still pretty unusual, a great patient-provider relationship also makes space for conversations about sexual pleasure and sexual behaviors.

>> **STI treatment and prevention:** You should be able to rely on your healthcare provider for information about and support with any STIs.

Exploring Mental and Emotional Health Resources

Transgender folks have higher rates of depression, anxiety, substance misuse, suicide, and suicidal thoughts due to the stigma, discrimination, and violence they face. This is a pretty serious health issue for many people, and it's important to remember that being trans or non-binary is not the cause.

If you're affected by mental and emotional health challenges, your PCP can be a great source of information, referrals, and support if you want help. The place where you get your transition care may also have a list of therapists, counselors, support groups, and online resources in your area. (See Chapter 12 for more info about reaching out for support and assistance.)

Inquiring about Your Provider's Level of Trans Education

It's perfectly legitimate to ask your healthcare providers how much training and experience they have in treating transgender and non-binary patients. Lack of experience doesn't have to be a deal-breaker — all trans medical experts have to start with their first non-binary or transgender patient at some point. But it can be a good sign if your provider has sought out training in this area, because it still isn't part of the standard curriculum in medical or nursing school. When medical professionals go out of their way to inform themselves about trans people, it almost always makes them more capable and confident.

Saying No

The MD on our writing team had this final thought about communicating with your healthcare provider: You should feel that you're able to say no to anything you're not comfortable talking about or doing. And if you feel uncomfortable more than you feel comfortable, you should feel empowered to find another provider. Your autonomy, agency, safety, and dignity must be preserved and protected by your medical practitioner.

Chapter 16

Ten (or So) Trans-Friendly Organizations

Although the United States still has a huge need for more resources for transgender and non-binary people, quite a few really great organizations are currently doing work that you need to know about.

In this chapter, you open a window onto ten or so (we couldn't help but include a few more) different groups that do a wonderful job advocating for transgender and non-binary people.

Advocates for Trans Equality

Advocates for Trans Equality (A4TE) is the foremost legal and lobbying group for the transgender community in the United States. In 2024, the Transgender Legal Defense and Education Fund and the National Center for Transgender Equality came together to combine their resources and impact, and formed A4TE.

They are one of the groups, along with the American Civil Liberties Union (ACLU), that files lawsuits on behalf of trans and non-binary people to help define their legal rights through the courts. They also lobby at the federal level to oppose dangerous federal law and to craft proactive and protective laws.

The ID documents center on A4TE's website covers every state and federal ID document, and what's required to change them. And A4TE is the organization that administers the single biggest survey of trans and non-binary people, the U.S. Transgender Survey.

You can find out more about all this and other work they do on their website (https://transequality.org/).

Transgender Resource Center of New Mexico

Transgender Resource Center of New Mexico (TGRCNM) has been around since 2007, and since then has grown to become a very effective, truly statewide organization. TGRCNM exists solely to serve transgender and non-binary New Mexicans, as well as their families and loved ones, through a combination of direct services, advocacy, and education.

The organization's services help folks with a range of needs, including emergency financial assistance; name changes; trans-specific items like binders and breast forms; a comprehensive Provider Directory on the website (https://tgrcnm.org/); a drop-in center where folks can get food, take a shower, do laundry, and more; a transitional living program; specific youth services; and so much more.

TGRCNM's advocacy includes policy work with businesses, medical clinics, and groups all over New Mexico to improve their trans policy and/or materials and make them more inclusive. The group has also worked with close partners at Equality New Mexico to change state law by, for example, updating the birth certificate law in 2019 to eliminate the surgical requirement and add the X marker, and revising the name change law in 2023 to eliminate the publication requirement.

Finally, TGRCNM delivers high-quality education about transgender and non-binary people to groups around New Mexico and throughout the United States. The organization has provided training to more than 4,000 groups since 2008, to amazing reviews.

Sylvia Rivera Law Project

Sylvia Rivera Law Project (SRLP) is a legal organization in New York City formed in 2002. They provide direct legal representation to transgender, non-binary, gender-nonconforming, and *intersex* folks (see Chapter 1) who are incarcerated, immigrants, or even simply low-income people who need assistance with challenges ranging from fighting healthcare discrimination to getting ID documents.

SRLP also engages in community organizing with incarcerated trans people around New York City. They generally work to advocate for and with trans, non-binary, and intersex folks who have a lot of barriers to speaking out, but mainly to being heard. Check out their website (https://srlp.org/) for more information.

Transathlete.com

Transathlete.com was founded by Chris Mosier in 2013. Mosier was the first out trans athlete to compete in the Olympic Trials in his appropriate gender category, in 2020. He is a longtime educator and advocate for trans and non-binary athletes. As an affected person himself, he brings a ton of passion to trying to increase access for trans folks to the world of sports and athletic competition.

The site has a cool, short history of trans athletes and the Olympic Games. But primarily it's a great clearinghouse of resources and existing policies regarding trans athletic participation. The site includes well-organized and easy-to-access examples from all around the world.

If you're looking for information about trans and non-binary folks in sports, this is the place to start.

Transgender Gender-Variant & Intersex Justice Project

Transgender Gender-Variant & Intersex Justice Project (TGIJP) became a formal organization in 2004 based on their existing work to support and assist trans, non-binary, and intersex folks in facilities of incarceration throughout California. Miss Major Griffin-Gracy, an incredible trans activist, was the first executive director of TGIJP. They began by providing legal services to trans and non-binary people, and now have programs in the areas of prison correspondence, reentry, leadership development, policy and budget advocacy, and housing.

TGIJP has always been led by trans women of color, and they embody what it means to be an agency run by and for vulnerable trans and non-binary folks. Their website (https://tgijp.org/) is the place to go to find out more about them, get connected to their work, and make a donation.

Transgender Law Center

Transgender Law Center (TLC) has been around since 2002, working for transgender and non-binary people through impact litigation, national organizing, and grant making.

The history-making National Center for Lesbian Rights fiscally sponsored TLC as a program in the beginning, until they became an independent nonprofit in 2004. TLC has been involved in some precedent-setting legal cases and continues to litigate cases that make a difference for trans communities.

TLC's leadership development focuses on empowering trans folks of color, and in 2024 they announced the Action for Transformation Fund, a partnership with rapid-response grantmaker Emergent Fund to move $1 million to "trans-led organizing, healing, and power-building efforts" (https://tinyurl.com/4a8h8me2).

In 2015 TLC promoted Kris Hayashi to executive director (ED), making him the first transgender person of color to lead a trans-specific organization the size of TLC. Then, in 2023, Shelby Chestnut took over the ED role. Chestnut is descended from the Assiniboine tribe of Montana, which means they're the first Native American ED at TLC and one of the first to be in the top leadership position of an LGBTQ organization.

TLC is out there doing the work every day, and you can find out more at https://transgenderlawcenter.org/.

Camp Lost Boys

Rocco Kayiatos is a transgender man, artist, and musician who gained early prominence as a rapper with the stage name Katastrophe, and who released albums in the 2000s. Along with Amos Mac, he founded the magazine *Original Plumbing* (a reference to trans guys who don't have bottom surgery — see Chapter 9). Over ten years, they released 20 issues of their groundbreaking magazine featuring trans men and focusing on trans male culture. Kayiatos is currently chief content officer at FOLX Health (you can find references to FOLX throughout this book), and the cocreator and director of the powerful and innovative program Camp Lost Boys.

The camp is an incredible chance for transgender men to experience the joy of summer sleepaway camp, which may not be something these folks had access to in their childhood. Some transgender men got to attend camp as kids, but they had to do it while being perceived as girls. Each camp is different, but some activities they offer include archery, ropes courses, hiking, and paintball. Their website, where you can get more information, register for camp, and join the mailing list, can be found at https://www.camplostboys.org/.

Trans Justice Funding Project

The Trans Justice Funding Project (TJFP) was created in 2012 by Gabriel Foster and Karen Pittelman in response to a dire need for funding for trans-led grassroots groups and efforts. Although trans communities have always engaged in mutual aid, community safety, and organizing, mainstream funding often is based on structures that lock some people and groups out.

Even the requirement to be a 501(c)(3) charitable organization is a big barrier for small or newly formed groups that may be doing transformational work in their communities.

TJFP employs only trans folks of color. They raise the money that funds their efforts directly from the communities they serve, and work to distribute it in an efficient, low-barrier manner.

Just eliminating the 501(c)(3) requirement to apply for funding through TJFP means that some emerging groups have gotten their start here. To apply for funding, donate, join the mailing list, or find out more, check out their website (https://www.transjusticefundingproject.org/).

TransLatin@ Coalition

Activist Bamby Salcedo founded the TransLatin@ Coalition in 2009 to provide advocacy and direct services to Latina transgender women who are immigrants to the United States. They are a chapter organization with offices in Houston, Atlanta, Chicago, and other U.S. cities.

TransLatin@ Coalition's Los Angeles chapter has a big presence in Southern California, with services that include economic development, legal assistance, transitional housing, and a drop-in center. Their annual GARRAS fashion show is a major event in LA.

You can find more info about this unique organization on their website (https://www.translatinacoalition.org/).

Notable Medical Organizations

These transgender organizations are specifically medical in nature. Around the country, some important transgender medical groups include

>> Fenway Health in Boston (https://fenwayhealth.org/)

>> University of California San Francisco Center of Excellence for Transgender Health (https://prevention.ucsf.edu/transhealth)

>> Callen-Lorde in New York City (https://callen-lorde.org/)

>> Howard Brown Health in Chicago (https://howardbrown.org/)

Honorable Mention

Our honorable mention category is for groups that do some really good work for transgender and non-binary people but aren't transgender-led or even necessarily transgender-focused.

Some highlights in this category are

>> Planned Parenthood (https://www.plannedparenthood.org/)

>> ACLU (https://www.aclu.org/)

>> PFLAG, formerly known as Parents and Friends of Lesbians and Gays (https://pflag.org/)

>> GLAAD (https://glaad.org/)

>> National LGBTQ Task Force (https://www.thetaskforce.org/)

>> GLSEN (https://www.glsen.org/)

Chapter **17**

Ten Ways to Support Transgender and Non-Binary People

Hopefully, as you come out and embark on your transition journey, you have family, friends, coworkers, or classmates who want to know how to help and support you. In this chapter, you get a peek at the advice the education team at Transgender Resource Center of New Mexico (TGRCNM) offers to *cisgender* folks (whose sex and gender match) around New Mexico, and throughout the United States, about how to be a good friend (or ally) to trans and non-binary people. So, arm your boosters with these ten important tips.

Educating Yourself

Asking questions of your trans or non-binary friend, neighbor, or family member is tempting, because they're right there. But to be a great ally, you have to independently seek out more information about transgender and non-binary folks. For example, TGRCNM provides in-person training on transgender issues day in and day out, along with support groups and volunteer opportunities. You may not have a similar resource near you, but you can turn to a few good options online.

Here are a couple of cool tools to get you started:

>> The Trans 101 guide from Advocates for Trans Equality (https://transequality.org/trans-101)

>> The Here We Are campaign (https://www.herewearenow.com/)

Respecting Names and Pronouns

It gets talked about so much that it starts to seem like the be-all and end-all of being a supporter of trans people. Using folks' correct names and pronouns is definitely not where being an ally stops. But it's absolutely where it begins.

TGRCNM points people to these two resources to show how profound correct name and pronoun use is:

>> A survey on the mental health benefits of using a young transgender person's chosen name (https://pmc.ncbi.nlm.nih.gov/articles/PMC6165713/)

>> The Trevor Project's 2021 National Survey on LGBTQ Youth Mental Health (https://www.thetrevorproject.org/survey-2021/)

According to the data, proper name and pronoun use has been shown to reduce suicidal behavior in trans and non-binary youth by as much as 56 percent. Both the survey and the study focus on trans youth, but calling people what they want to be called doesn't have any age limits.

Helping with Bathroom Access

As far-fetched as it may sound if you don't have to deal with this problem, your trans and non-binary friends may really appreciate you offering to help them go to the bathroom if they ever need it. You can accompany someone to the bathroom if you use the same one they do. Or, you can stand outside and prevent other people from entering while your friend uses the bathroom in peace.

You can also make bathrooms safer in any setting where you spend a lot of time. For example, bathrooms with multiple stalls and gender designations should have signage that reassures and welcomes trans and non-binary folks who need to go. You can reach out to management at your job, school, house of worship, or recreational center and go to bat for adding inclusive signs. A guide from the Rainbow Alliance Inclusion Network in Washington state offers some great suggestions (https://tinyurl.com/3wx4abu5).

Making Sure You Don't Out Someone

A lot of trans and non-binary folks have trouble, at least some of the time, correcting people who refer to them by the wrong name and pronouns. So, they may really appreciate you stepping in to help. For instance, if you're at a coffee shop, and the barista calls your trans masculine friend "she," you can gently say, "Oh, I think you mean *he*. My friend is *he*." This may mean more than you'll ever know to someone you care about who is trans.

At the same time, you have to be aware of who knows your friend's correct name and pronouns. Some people are out at work but not to their parents. Others are out in almost every setting but may still have one space in their life where they feel they have to hold back their truth. If you have a trans friend you want to support, make sure to ask if there's any place they *don't* want you to use their chosen name and correct pronouns. Then you can step in and help with confidence.

Offering Your Pronouns

In the old days of 2008 or so, we used to encourage cisgender folks to ask if they weren't sure of someone's pronouns. These days, this seems like poor advice. If you just walk up and ask someone their pronouns, you may as well say, "You look odd to me, and I'm not sure how to speak about you." Plus, once you understand more about non-binary people, the advantages of everyone putting their pronouns out there become clearer. The expectation can't be that only the gender variant people have to specify their pronouns. That won't ever work, since there's no way to tell who is gender variant from the outside. When you put your pronouns out there, you are helping this to become standard operating procedure, which it needs to be!

Non-binary people, who don't feel like a man or a woman, can embrace a stereotypically masculine or feminine appearance. Anyone you meet may be non-binary, no matter how stereotypically male or female they look. Turn one more corner in your mind, and you realize that *you* could be non-binary. Not that you are.

If you are a man or a woman, so are many transgender people. But your binary gender being a core part of your identity, something you know deeply and truly, isn't a trait people can see on the outside. Even if you have a beard, love wearing makeup and dresses, or are proudly bald, that isn't enough evidence for a stranger to know your gender and pronouns, because non-binary people sport all those looks, too.

You can show a high level of cultural fluency by offering your pronouns in

TIP

>> Verbal introductions

You can try a variation of "Hi, I'm Adrien and I use 'he' pronouns. I'm the director of education at TGRCNM."

>> Email signatures

>> Virtual meeting platform captions

>> Name tags

>> Business cards

>> Social media bios

>> A pin or button on your lapel or lanyard at work

Teaching Kids about LGBTQ People

LGBTQ people have always existed, and their existence isn't sexual or controversial by nature. If you're a cisgender person, and also someone who is helping raise a child or children, it's important to make sure that your kids know about LGBTQ people, their stories, and their contributions.

Hopefully, you have LGBTQ folks in your family or social circles. If so, be open about their identities with your kiddos. Not only can your kids *be* transgender or non-binary, but they will definitely know folks who are. Being open about all the different kinds of people in the world your kids may interact with in a variety of ways is one of the key ingredients to inoculating them against prejudice.

GLSEN, an organization intent on ending discrimination in education, has some great lesson plans and other cool resources that may inspire parents to talk to their children about famous or important transgender and non-binary people throughout history (https://www.glsen.org/resources/educator-resources).

Using Gender-Neutral Language

At the beginning of this chapter we provide a couple of links to data showing that correct name and pronoun usage is literally suicide prevention (see the earlier section "Educating Yourself"). While that may be hard for a cisgender person to relate to, it still illustrates how powerful language can be.

A 2019 article in the *Guardian* (https://tinyurl.com/yc2nvwac) cited a study that concluded that the use of "language that actively includes women and LGBT people . . . makes a real difference in reducing gender stereotyping." According to a researcher quoted in the article, "Using gender-neutral language is a positive step towards creating a world where everyone is accepted without exception."

Even if you're open to using gender-neutral language, though, how do you change a lifetime of habits? The following online articles can help you get started:

>> Grammarly's tips on using gender-neutral language (https://www.grammarly.com/blog/language-trends-culture/gender-neutral-language/)

>> A Planned Parenthood "Ask the Experts" column (https://tinyurl.com/2r4jterc)

>> An amazing guide from a really cool website (https://tinyurl.com/56vkaxf5)

Working Through Challenging Feelings with Others

When someone in your life comes out as transgender or non-binary and begins their transition journey, you may have a complex mix of feelings. There's nothing wrong with that, and you aren't alone. An online or in-person support group for parents and family members of transgender and non-binary people can offer a nonjudgmental, caring space to work through any grief, anger, sadness, surprise, disappointment, or resentment you may have.

Giving voice to your feelings, especially when you're sharing them with folks who understand or even relate to your emotions, can be healing. Talking with others is a great way to shift and eventually transform your negative feelings. You can also get answers and maybe some peace of mind by reading an article about transgender children on the Human Rights Campaign's website (https://tinyurl.com/ye9hd28y).

REMEMBER

You can find many good options for discovering more about transgender and non-binary people and processing your feelings, but one of them is not the trans or non-binary person in your life. It's too difficult for them to hold space for your negative feelings, and it's a real challenge to understand that your reaction is just an emotional outpouring and not a real response to who they are. Even if your trans loved one or friend says they're okay with being your counselor, they're really not the best choice.

Speaking Up through Advocacy

Because you may be only indirectly affected by all the issues facing trans and non-binary folks, it can sometimes feel less risky for you to be the person who steps in to say something. You can speak up for transgender and non-binary people in many settings, and your advocacy can be anything from interrupting misgendering, to asking your employer whether your workplace has transgender-inclusive health benefits. Advocates for Trans Equality (A4TE) has an online guide with many good ideas for how to help (https://tinyurl.com/38kkcnz4).

Find out if you have any local or statewide trans organizations and join their mailing lists or make a donation. Even if your contribution is small, they'll appreciate it! Check out national trans advocacy groups, of which A4TE is foremost. Jump in when it's time to email your congressperson or testify before your state legislature. Transgender and non-binary people are a minority group and will never achieve full equality without the support of their families, loved ones, friends, and allies.

Showing Visible Support

It means a lot to transgender and non-binary people when cisgender individuals show their support with outward gestures and signs. What does this mean? Here are some ways to show your love for trans communities on the outside:

>> **Patches:** You can attach pro-trans slogans and graphic patches to your clothes or backpack.

>> **Pins/buttons:** From declaring your own pronouns, to urging people to "Support Trans Rights," these badges convey that you're a safe and supportive person.

>> **Posters:** You can find pro-trans posters at online retailers like Zazzle and Redbubble. Some are serious, and some are cute and funny.

>> **Stickers:** Put supportive stickers on your computer, car, water bottle — wherever you have space for them!

>> **T-shirts:** Search online for websites like TeePublic, which has a large selection of trans tees (`https://www.teepublic.com/t-shirts?query=transgender`).

REMEMBER

Don't forget that the discrimination and violence trans people face isn't evenly distributed — it's *intersectional*. That means that if a trans or non-binary person has other marginalized characteristics, they're more likely to experience bad outcomes. Data from the 2022 U.S. Transgender Survey shows clearly that folks who are trans and disabled, undocumented, neurodivergent, unhoused, women/femme, and/or people of color (especially Black and Indigenous people) often have significantly worse experiences of stigma, discrimination. and violence. So, you don't have to restrict your support to just the trans aspect of someone's identity.

This chapter provides some guidance on how you can support trans and non-binary people. What else can you think of?

Index

A

A4TE (Advocates for Trans Equality), 41, 53, 55, 72, 76, 77, 179, 209–210, 220
AAP (American Academy of Pediatrics), 20
ace. *See* asexual
ACEs (adverse childhood experiences), 103–104
ACLU, 214
acne, as a risk of masculinizing hormones, 124
activity, as a consideration for clothing, 61
acupuncture, 190
Adam's apple, facial feminizing surgery (FFS) and, 146
adoption, 170–171
advance directives, creating, 88–89
adverse childhood experiences (ACEs), 103–104
Advocates for Trans Equality (A4TE), 41, 53, 55, 72, 76, 77, 179, 209–210, 220
advocating, 220
aesthetic only packers, 64
aesthetics, 96, 109–113
Affordable Care Act (2010), 205
age
  as a consideration for clothing, 61
  voice and, 157
agency adoption, 170
agender, 10
Alexander, Bruce, 156
allostatic loads, 95
ALT (anterolateral thigh) flap, for phalloplasty, 141
American Academy of Dermatology, 63
American Academy of Family Physicians, 97
American Academy of Pediatrics (AAP), 20
American Bar Association, 85
American Dental Association, 111
American Psychiatric Association (APA), 18, 100
American Psychological Association (APA), 21
American Speech-Language-Hearing Association, 159
Ancestry.com, 169
anchor, as a type of top surgery, 137–138

Anderson, Lucy Hicks, 200
androgynous, 45
anesthesia complications, from bottom surgery, 143, 150
animal therapy, 108, 190
anterolateral thigh (ALT) flap, for phalloplasty, 141
antiandrogen, 148
anticipating changes/timelines, 118–120, 124–127
APA (American Psychiatric Association), 18, 100
APA (American Psychological Association), 21
appearance. *See* style and appearance
areolas, 138
art therapy, 108, 190
articulation, for voices, 156
ASCVD (atherosclerotic cardiovascular disease) risk score, 97
asexual, 12–13, 48
atherosclerotic cardiovascular disease (ASCVD) risk score, 97
Aunt Flow, 112
Ávila, Amelio Robles, 200

B

bathroom access, 27, 216–217
batwing, as a type of top surgery, 138
behavioral health resources, 189–192
"Bending the Mold" guide, 55
Beyond the Gender Binary (Vaid-Menon), 199
bilateral mastectomy, 137
bilateral stimulation, 190
binding, 26–27, 67–69
biological sex, 11
birth certificates, getting new, 76
bisexual, 12–13, 48
Blac, Jecca (makeup artist), 62
BlackLine, 193
bleeding, as a complication of bottom surgery, 143, 150
blood work, baseline, 117

libido
about, 206
decreased, from feminizing hormones, 125
defined, 47–48, 205
increased, from masculinizing hormones, 119
lidocaine, 110
life implications, of gender transition, 16–17
life-sustaining options, in advance directives, 88
lips, facial feminizing surgery (FFS) and, 146–147
living will. *See* advance directives
location, for therapists and health care providers, 187
logistics, 99
long-term commitments, of gender transition, 48–55
Lost Connections (Hari), 105
low-disclosure life, 55
lowering risk of mental health issues, 189

M

Making Queer History, 200
male-pattern baldness, from masculinizing hormones, 119
managing
clothing changes, 59–64
grooming changes, 59–64
personal questions, 40–41
relationships, 49–51
trauma for trans and non-binary youth, 108–109
unsupportive people, 43–45
mannerisms, shifting, 26
MAP (Movement Advancement Project), 74–75
masculinizing hormones
about, 118
anticipating changes and timelines, 118–120
choosing delivery methods, 121–122
determining doses, 122–123
risks of, 123–124
masculinizing surgery
about, 136
bottom surgery, 140–145
top surgery, 136–140
masculinizing voices, 161–163
massage, 190

Maté, Gabor, 104, 156
The Matrix (film), 200
McBride, Sarah (activist)
Tomorrow Will Be Different, 199
medialization laryngoplasty, 164
Medicaid, 99, 159
medical cannabis, 108
medical organizations, 214
medical power of attorney, 87
medical transition
about, 30–31
detransitioning, 34–35
physical changes, 32–34
treatment, therapy, and ongoing care, 31–32
meditation, 190–191
Meetup, 40, 182
meet-ups, 21
menstruation
about, 112–113
interruption of, from masculinizing hormones, 119–120
mental health
criteria for gender dysphoria, 117
evaluating, 117
resources for, 206
support for
about, 185
behavioral health resources, 189–192
finding care, 185–188
lowering risks of issues, 189
suicide prevention resources, 192–194
types of counseling, 188
metoidioplasty, 140–141
microdosing, 131
military records, modifying, 78–80
mindfulness, for trauma, 109
misgendering, 27
MLD (musculocutaneous latissimus dorsi) flap, for phalloplasty, 141
modifying
body profile, 64–70
immigration documents, 80–81
military records, 78–80

Y

About the Authors

Adrien Lawyer cofounded the Transgender Resource Center of New Mexico (TGRCNM) in 2007 to provide services, education, and advocacy for the transgender community. **T. Michael Trimm** serves as the executive director at TGRCNM, and **Erik Wolf** is the organization's director of operations. **Molly McClain**, MD, MPH, MS, is a board-certified family and community medicine physician who has provided gender care for people of all ages in New Mexico for many years.

Acknowledgments

The author team would like to acknowledge all the TGRCNM participants and community, who remind us why our work is important and our existence is valued. The incredible team at Wiley literally made this book possible. Thanks to Tracy and Kelly and all the folks who helped shape and sculpt *Gender Transition For Dummies* into the book you're holding.

Adrien thanks his spouse, Shari, and kid, Sam, who are the foundation of everything he does. He also must shout out a big thank-you to his "brother," Zane, the cofounder of TGRCNM, and his "sister," Carmela, a true friend and the invaluable brain behind Chapter 6.

Michael would like to acknowledge his father, who was the first family member to accept, support, and defend him in his transition.

Erik would like to acknowledge his Aunt Kristal, whose steadfast support and guidance made him the person he is today.

We dedicate this book to all the trans, non-binary, and gender-expansive people who have been lost to violence (both structural and interpersonal), societal and familial disconnection, and loneliness. We also dedicate this book to all the trans, non-binary, and gender-expansive people whose lives and work have allowed us to live more authentically. Their journeys continue to inspire, giving hope and courage to many. We hope this book is a beacon for some of our community members who are looking for their way home.

Publisher's Acknowledgments

Senior Acquisitions Editor: Jennifer Yee
Managing Editor: Sofia Malik
Project Manager: Tracy Brown Hamilton
Copy Editor: Kelly Brillhart

Production Editor: Saikarthick Kumarasamy
Cover Image: © Mappleford/Shutterstock

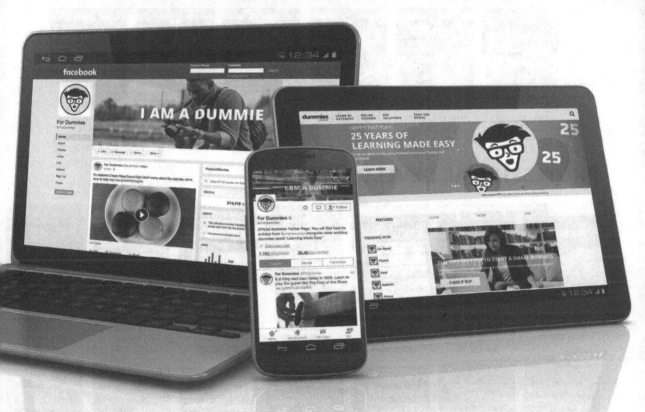
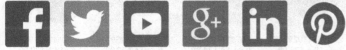
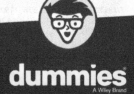

PERSONAL ENRICHMENT

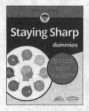
Staying Sharp
9781119187790
USA $26.00
CAN $31.99
UK £19.99

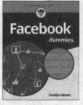
Facebook
9781119179030
USA $21.99
CAN $25.99
UK £16.99

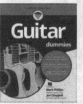
Guitar
9781119293354
USA $24.99
CAN $29.99
UK £17.99

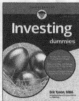
Investing
9781119293347
USA $22.99
CAN $27.99
UK £16.99

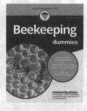
Beekeeping
9781119310068
USA $22.99
CAN $27.99
UK £16.99

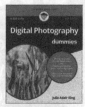
Digital Photography
9781119235606
USA $24.99
CAN $29.99
UK £17.99

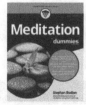
Meditation
9781119251163
USA $24.99
CAN $29.99
UK £17.99

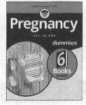
Pregnancy
9781119235491
USA $26.99
CAN $31.99
UK £19.99

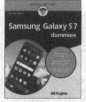
Samsung Galaxy S7
9781119279952
USA $24.99
CAN $29.99
UK £17.99

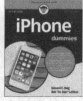
iPhone
9781119283133
USA $24.99
CAN $29.99
UK £17.99

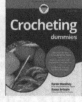
Crocheting
9781119287117
USA $24.99
CAN $29.99
UK £16.99

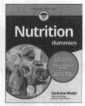
Nutrition
9781119130246
USA $22.99
CAN $27.99
UK £16.99

PROFESSIONAL DEVELOPMENT

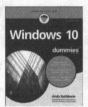
Windows 10
9781119311041
USA $24.99
CAN $29.99
UK £17.99

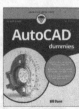
AutoCAD
9781119255796
USA $39.99
CAN $47.99
UK £27.99

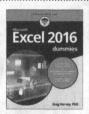
Excel 2016
9781119293439
USA $26.99
CAN $31.99
UK £19.99

QuickBooks 2017
9781119281467
USA $26.99
CAN $31.99
UK £19.99

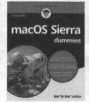
macOS Sierra
9781119280651
USA $29.99
CAN $35.99
UK £21.99

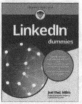
LinkedIn
9781119251132
USA $24.99
CAN $29.99
UK £17.99

Windows 10
9781119310563
USA $34.00
CAN $41.99
UK £24.99

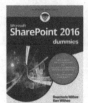
SharePoint 2016
9781119181705
USA $29.99
CAN $35.99
UK £21.99

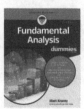
Fundamental Analysis
9781119263593
USA $26.99
CAN $31.99
UK £19.99

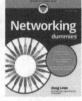
Networking
9781119257769
USA $29.99
CAN $35.99
UK £21.99

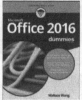
Office 2016
9781119293477
USA $26.99
CAN $31.99
UK £19.99

Office 365
9781119265313
USA $24.99
CAN $29.99
UK £17.99

Salesforce.com
9781119239314
USA $29.99
CAN $35.99
UK £21.99

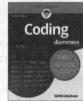
Coding
9781119293323
USA $29.99
CAN $35.99
UK £21.99

dummies.com

dummies
A Wiley Brand